MW01284096

A Hidden Killer: Amniotic Fluid Embolism

羊水栓塞

An Ob-Gyn's Experience

Bitao Lian, A.P., Ob-Gyn (China)

练碧涛

PRAISE FOR THE AUTHOR

This is an important book about AFE, a rare and usually fatal condition in which amniotic fluid suddenly floods the body of a woman giving birth. It has been known to cause afflicted women to commit suicide and in at least one case a husband left behind to go mad.

Dr. Lian hopes that by sharing her knowledge of AFE and its treatment, both with the medical profession and with the rest of us, she can save lives that could otherwise be lost. And, I think because this is a personal crusade, she begins in the poetic present, on the coast of Florida, flashes back to vivid descriptions of cases she encountered while practicing as an Ob-Gyn in China, then goes on to other cases she has researched to learn more about this silent killer of women.

Once she has described the disease and its consequences—in one part of the world it is called "death"—she turns to prevention, offering pregnant women advice on how to take care of themselves to minimize their chances of being struck down. She also describes the symptoms they should immediately tell their doctors about if they encounter them in the birthing process. Then, she tells medical practitioners how to diagnose AFE as early as possible—emphasizing the fact that if this condition is present, time is of the essence—and advises them to "treat first, test later." She follows that with highly specific information about the treatment procedures she believes are most likely to save the lives of women and their fetuses. She even has a list of conditions that may be misdiagnosed as AFE.

Finally, Dr. Lian offers us a fascinating chapter about the *Mona Lisa*, in which she suggests that Leonardo da Vinci may have understood this condition over five hundred years before anyone else.

In sum, I found this book both moving and useful, and, if it gets the audience it deserves, I really believe Dr. Lian will in fact have saved lives.

—Lola Haskins, American Poet

Bitao Lian

Copyright 2018 by Bi Tao Lian

All rights reserved.

No part of this publication may be
reproduced, stored in a retrieval
system, or transmitted in any form
or by any means, electronic, mechanical,
photocopying, recording, or
otherwise, without the prior
permission of the author.

ISBN: 9781980509882

DEDICATION

To mothers all over the world

CONTENTS

ABOUT THE AUTHOR

BI TAO LIAN WAS born in 1962 in Zijin County, Guangdong Province, China. She was admitted to Guangzhou Medical University in 1978, where she received training for five years. She graduated in August 1983, and then she was assigned by the government to Shenzhen City Central Hospital in Guangdong Province, as a obstetrician and gynecologist. In 1986, she was assigned to the First Affiliated Hospital of Zhongsan Medical University for a year of obstetrics and gynecology. In 1990, she moved to Sydney, Australia, to study at the College of Natural Therapeutics. She also worked as a Chinese medicine practitioner at Sydney's Chinese Herbs Medical Center. In 1992, she emigrated to Florida, in the United States, where, during the following year, she obtained an American Acupuncture Practitioner's license and subsequently opened her clinic, the Oriental Healing Center. In 2000, Dr. Lian was invited by Kevin B. Kern, M.D., and James T. Menges, M.D., to the Pain Clinic at the Department of Veterans Affairs Medical Center, Gainesville, Florida. This clinic was conducted with Chinese medicine practitioners in Western medicine and demonstrated the remarkable pain-relief effect possible with acupuncture. Previously, in 1997, former First Lady Nancy Reagan helped organize a detoxification program using nontraditional treatment, including acupuncture, and fully acknowledged the efficacy of traditional Chinese medicine.

PREFACE

序言

MY LIFE BEGAN WITH a first cry in March 1962, in Zijin County, Guangdong Province, China, at the time of year when peach trees were in blossom, in a land that long ago was dominated by dinosaurs. It is the farmland area that adhered to the Central Plains Hakka culture of family Chinese medicine practice. My great-grandfather was a well-known local Chinese medicine practitioner who used specials skills with his hands to fix fractured bone; he was an expert at treating disease with acupuncture and herbs, and he cured many patients. My kind, honest grandfather DeTang Zheng completed a few years of private school, gained an understanding of Chinese herbal medicine, and began practicing medicine in the country. Thanks to his master, Mr. Cai, he learned and mastered the use of dozens of Chinese medicine–formulated ointments and cured many cervical lymphadenopathies and tuberculoses. Another significant result of his practice was that he shared his knowledge with me. He treated one patient at a time, and his fee was one Yuan. He bought a piece of land in the center of the county and, getting up early and going home late, worked hard with my grandmother Mei Chen, cutting down trees from the hillside and using them as pillars to support the roof of the home and the practice he built. They used the local yellow-clay mud to form the walls and floors. The result of their efforts was a three-story Hakka-style compound with front and rear halls, which would become for them and for younger generations both a shelter and a warm and happy home.

My father, Tie Qiang Lian, was the person I respected most in my life. He was a local official who led by example. He worked diligently at his job, often slept little, and spared no effort in working for the people—like a spring silkworm will work at producing silk until its death. Unfortunately, he died of liver cancer. Before his death, he said his last words to me—his daughter, the doctor. It was his wish "to donate my cornea to a patient who needs it." However, because he had hepatitis C as a result of a heart-surgery transfusion, he was not able to give his gift of love to the world. My mother, Yanlan Zheng, is strong, diligent, and economical—a typical Hakka woman—and always works, as the saying goes, "at being like the mother hen who does her utmost to take care of her children!"

Since beginning primary school, I have insisted on keeping a daily diary. I was a Marxist-Leninist activist in high school, and my diary was selected by my teacher to be included in the newspaper column of Zijin Middle School. Because of my persistent habit of writing diaries, I can describe what happened every day of my life. Thus, what I have written in this book is not a fictional creation but rather consists of descriptions of actual events.

In 1978, China welcomed reform and an "opening up" and resumed its second year of giving college entrance examinations. The same year, I graduated from high school, passed the country's examinations, and was admitted to the Guangzhou Medical University. I was the only female student in Zijin County to be admitted at the provincial level to the university. During my five years studying at the university, I did my best to gain medical knowledge, taking little or no time for entertainment or romance. I only wanted to learn about medicine, to become a good doctor, to cure patients, and to educate people. On August 13, 1983, I graduated with honors and was soon assigned to Shenzhen City Central Hospital as a gynecologist. As a member of the Chinese National Obstetrics and Gynecology staff and an energetic 21-year-old young woman, I was devoted to saving lives and welcoming the heavy workload associated with childbirth, while participating in China's national prosperity. That year, Shenzhen was a new and special economic zone under President Xiaoping Deng's leadership in reform and opening up. The place was full of vigor, vitality, and dust. "Time is money; speed is life!" was the slogan of the times. Many young entrepreneurs gathered there to acquire earthly possessions and help create a new era. Such young cities were full of young couples, and the fertility rates were extra-high.

In 1984, more than 500 newborns were de-livered each month at the Central Hospital. A doctor diagnosed and treated 60 patients daily in the outpatient department. At the clinic each day, the waiting room was full. The many waiting pa-tients were as noisy as a swarm of buzzing bees. They filed in one by one for my treatment, and when I needed to use the toilet, I had to run to it. Twenty-four beds per doctor were managed in the inpatient department, and doctors often worked day and night. At the height of my work there, I was delivering nine babies per night and performing six operations per day.

Sometimes, after 24 hours on the night shift, I went back to my dorm, fell asleep, and even failed to wash my feet, which were streaked with blood from the new mothers during their deliveries. Often I awoke confused, not knowing whether it was dusk or dawn. The work intensity was like being in a war zone. With the change of pace in China that resulted from the reform, I was one of the pioneers in Shenzhen participating in the reconstruction, and I devoted all my time and youth to work. Living in a new city building was a reward I felt I deserved. I spent six and a half days a week in the hospital (I also had to return to hospital rounds on Sundays) and did five-day rotations of 24-hour night shifts. I was young and energetic, not afraid of suffering, and not afraid of working hard or of being tired, and I felt life was full of hope and sunshine.

I knew that "water can carry a boat," as the old saying goes. I had been given the water-related name of my father (Bi Tao), and I believe I very naturally understood that amniotic fluid is the source of life. I also believe I am a rare person who has witnessed the first, most primitive stage of amniotic fluid. It happened on the morning of New Year's Day in 1983 when I operated on a patient who was 43 days pregnant and who unfortunately had an ectopic pregnancy. After opening her abdominal cavity, I saw a wonderful, unforgettable image of life: In the patient's left fallopian-tube ampulla I saw a growing embryo of about 0.8 centimeters in diameter, similar in form to the crystal orb Jesus holds in his left hand in Leonardo da Vinci's painting *Salvator Mundi (Savior of the World)*. In the middle of the ampulla was a reddish heart beating regularly, surrounded by crystal-clear amniotic fluid. The mung bean–sized orb looked similar to a fairy-land, with a most beautiful being there in its early state. The surrounding fluid would have been the first swimming pool for this being. In all our lives it is a first swimming pool for each of us, the world's purest swimming pool, where one can be nourished by lassi. It is a beautiful world that nurtures life, and it is also a source of life. I gazed at the wonderful being for what seemed like a long time, as I was unwilling to pick up the scalpel. Today I still regret not having a video recorder in the operating room with which to record an image of this rare being. Also I lament that medical treatment at that time did not allow for transplanting an embryo into a uterus, in order that the life may have continued growing.

On one occasion, I experienced the taste of amniotic fluid. It happened on a winter evening in 1988 when I became involved in an emergency delivery of a baby inside a car. The infant was pale and not breathing; the situation was urgent. No suction pump or any other medical equipment was available, so I held the baby in my arms and used a mouth-to-mouth method to clear the amniotic fluid and secretions from its airway, disregarding possible infectious disease. I sucked and spat, sucked and spat, until the newborn issued a crisp crying sound. Amniotic fluid entered my esophagus and then my stomach, causing bursts of burning. Unfortunately for me, the fluid tasted salty and fishy, and its unbearably rancid taste has been unforgettable.

"Water can also carry a capsized boat," as I learned. After my first two years of work, I met a hidden killer called amniotic fluid embolism (AFE), and it changed my life's trajectory. I sensed a river of endless time.

People's lives can differ so greatly. Some find paths that are easily accessible, while some find paths that are bumpy. Some people are prominent; some are dull; some are rich; some are poor. Some people have longevity, and some die prematurely. One thing seems constant: life is a process of dreaming. We all have our own wonderful dreams, and we weave, step by step, to achieve our goals, while working hard and struggling. I have now entered middle age, and my mood is peaceful. I now only want to do my best for my fellow human beings, for my patients, my family, and myself. Medicine combines science and humanity, and literature combines individuals and human nature. Whereas human nature is the soil of literature, humanity illuminates medicine. Decades of clinical experience is the soil of my writing, and I have worked hard at it, often in the dead of night, writing to both dissect myself and discover the nature of AFE. My family and friends have tried to persuade me not to write about sensitive domestic topics, such as the Mingjian Tian incident that I discuss in chapter 7, so that I might safely return to my hometown in the future. But my heart is bright, compassionate, and partnered with complex ideas. I wanted to learn from the famous doctor Qiaozhi Lin how to be a good obstetrician-gynecologist (Ob-Gyn). After my experiences with the merciless killer AFE, and after studying in Australia and opening a clinic in the US, I wanted to know much more.

It has been difficult for me to change my Chinese accent because I have so much nostalgia for my homeland. In recent years, it has worried me more, knowing that sometimes patients' family members insult or assault their doctors in China. After my long-term research and analysis of cases that presented in the Yu Lin City Central Hospital of Shanxi Province, I began to realize the necessity of educating others about the deadly disorder that has caused pregnant women to jump from buildings just before childbirth. In my spare time and during sleepless nights, I have discovered more about this strange disorder by striving to understand its origins and in urging that precautionary measures be taken. One of my missions as a doctor is to make everyone aware of AFE so that the great need for preventive measures will be understood. After publishing the Chinese version of this book, I translated it into English so that people all over the world would know more about it. It is my desire to have a Rongrong Ma Day set aside on every August 31, as a world day of prevention, which for me would be somewhat similar to the World Book Day observed on April 23. I encourage anyone who is able to add to my understanding of AFE to send their valuable comments! It is my sincere hope that encouragement and support will come from all corners of the earth and that this book will help my readers.

CHAPTER 1
After the Hurricane
飓风过后

IT WAS LATE AFTERNOON on September 17, 2017, after I had attended to a patient in St. Augustine, Florida, the oldest city in the US. (It is about 250 miles away, a four-hour drive, from US President Donald Trump's winter residence at the Mar-a-Lago Club in Palm Beach.) St. Augustine has experienced some of the strongest hurricanes in the history of the US, but I had not noticed that birds swirled over the ocean, indicating more violent storms to come. I saw only a few exquisite seagulls walking leisurely on the beach. However, the clear, blue ocean water had suddenly disappeared and was replaced by the appearance of a uterus with hypoxia and turbid, yellow amniotic water. This was one of Florida's most beautiful white beaches. Now the edge of it was splashed by yellow-white waves, which from a distance looked like flocculent, stranded jellyfish on the shoreline, reminding me of a uterine cavity and a baby's body with hair covered by mucus. Tide fluctuations, driven by the ocean breeze, formed crisscrossed mesh lines, which looked like the smooth muscle of the uterus, but even more choppy. The waves had lost their former gentleness and began to violently slap at the coast, tumbling in, wave after wave. As the water rushed onto the beach, it made me feel as if I were in a sea of Taijiquan. Suddenly, as I stood in the surf, a wave rushed over me, knocking me down and causing a finger of my left hand to strike against something hard. The sharp pain I felt was from the rocks on the beach that I had slammed against. I felt an inexplicable fear in my heart that chilled me. Distracted, I took three steps backward, as if a mysterious killer were lurking about me, attempting to drag me into the depths of the dark ocean. The urge to cry overcame me, and I quickly ran to the parking lot and got into my car, where I locked the door and prepared to drive home. When I looked back at the beach, I saw that the dark sky was clinging to the ocean and that together they seamlessly resembled the uterus of a full-term pregnant woman. My imagination and feelings were caused by an occupational condition typical for Ob-Gyns. I drove the car with my left hand holding onto the steering wheel and my right hand grasping my phone while I read the news and WeChat comments online. I read about major events at home and abroad and then saw the hot headline "Pregnant woman jumped from hospital window during the delivery process." I felt significantly worried by this news item and continued to read, despite the terrible darkness behind me, and I felt that I had to continue reading until I reached the conclusion.

CHAPTER 2
She Jumped From the Building with Her Fetus
茸茸跳楼

THE INCIDENT OCCURRED AT 8:13 p.m. on August 31, 2017, at the First Central Hospital of Yu Lin City, in Shanxi Province, China. A 27-year-old primiparous pregnant woman was on standby at the Suide District Hospital. At full-term, the fetus was dead. Prior to this, her cervix was nearly fully opened, but it seemed to her that her abdomen had a sharp, bursting pain she could no longer withstand, and she felt great irritability as a result. She had continued to beg the midwife for a cesarean section, and she rushed out of the waiting room several times and reportedly "got on her knees" to ask her husband and family to agree to the procedure.

During the previous few days, it was reported by the hospital that "a C-section had been proposed but rejected by the pregnant woman's husband." Details were given, indicating that both the family and the hospital had "refused C-section," each "preferring not to use the painless delivery method," and so on. At the same time, reports from newspapers and television shows and friends' discussions on WeChat had people guessing why she had given up her life. What had led a woman who likely would have been a happy mother to commit suicide? What had caused her to cast herself into the abyss? Did she have a death wish? Everything I read made my heart tremble. Had this hidden killer, which I had seen as a gynecologist and which had caused me to have nightmares, struck again? Of course, hospital rules and ethics are not always sound, and coupled with improper management, tragedies can occur. Both doctors and patients are victims, while the real and weird killer is ignored.

First of all, Rong Rong Ma, why did you jump? Some people in China even suspect that you were an alien belonging to an evolved species that is particularly afraid of pain.

The main indicators of a normal labor, regular uterine contractions, were sustained for more than 30 seconds intermittently for about 5 to 6 minutes and accompanied by progressive cervical-canal flattening, cervical dilatation, and fetal exposure. The labor contractions intermittently shortened to about every 2 to 3 minutes, at a longer duration of about 50 to 60 seconds and with increasing intensity to the cervix, which was nearly fully open. The uterine contractions came as often as every 1 minute at slightly longer durations of up to 1 minute or more. Normal physiological contractions are regular, paroxysmal, intermittent, and tolerable (although some women have painful lower-valve contractions).

According to the records of condition maintained by midwives Zhang Fan and Liu Li, the patient's pain, fury, and agitation were great. She was not being attended to by medical staff, but she resolutely requested a C-section. A camera showed that she left the childbirth center several times to let her husband, Zhuang Zhuang Yan, know about her pain. In her present state, she could not stand but knelt directly on the floor. Based on my experience in obstetrics and gynecology, I think her pain occurred because of

ankylosing uterine contraction, which is pathological pain. Unfortunately, the medical record
that the media published was incomplete. I called
the obstetrics and gynecology department of Yulin
City Hospital in Shaanxi Province at least ten
times to try to understand the situation and to
suggest that an autopsy and pathology examination be done and then repeated to determine
the true cause of her death. However, each time I
mentioned the patient's name, the staff immediately hung up the telephone. I could only gather
clues from the available information, make infer-
ences, and hope to find answers. No history of
mental illness or psychiatric drug use was noted.
During prenatal examination, a color B-mode
ultrasound scan showed that the fetal biparietal
diameter (BPD) was 9.90 cm; usually a full-term
fetal BPD is no more than 9.33 cm (at 40 weeks,
standard deviation of fetal BPD is 9.28 cm$\pm$0.05
cm). It has been suggested that the fetal head
was too large. If the doctor had found that to be
the case, progress in the labor most likely would
have been affected, as it would have been difficult for the woman to endure such pathological,
ankylosing pain, which likely would have resulted
in a ruptured uterus. The precursor was the
hidden embolism. When I saw the CCTV news
interview online, I noticed that Dr. Huo, Yulin City
Central Hospital's obstetrics and gynecology director, did not discuss C-section indications due to
cephalopelvic disproportion and the problem of
uterine rupture. The condition records did not
include blood pressure or heart rate measurements. How far apart had her contractions been,
and what were their duration and intensity,
especially during intravenous infusion of oxyto-

cin? The disorder was so hidden that even Ob-Gyns found it difficult to recognize its presence in her body. However, it quietly sneaked in. The amniotic fluid had flowed like hurricane-driven ocean water, pouring through her body, with influx into her lungs, heart, and brain, causing her uterus to be painfully torn apart like a ship at sea torn apart by two violent rip currents.

In fact, the patient had previously received an omen from her deadly enemy. The midwife's psychological counseling not only failed to solve her problem but also delayed treatment. Acting on survival instinct, the patient asked for a C-section, and in her desperation she left the delivery room several times to walk to the C-section waiting area. Amniotic fluid may have entered her blood circulation, resulting in severe pain, irritability, loss of consciousness, exhaustion, emotionalism, and an out-of-control state. Unbearable pain, fury, frustration, and helplessness led to her desperation. Misery caused her to jump from a window on the fifth floor of the hospital's childbirth center, along with her innocent baby—who had been with her for ten months and might have looked forward to life in this world.

The patient was a young woman (born in 1990) who had had a healthy body. She was a member of the communist party, and she had a bachelor's degree. She had longed for a better life and desired to advance in this world. The child in her uterus became part of the mysterious disorder. This mother became so miserable that she let go of her life and left her loved ones when in her prime. She had no chance to text a good-bye message to her husband, even with a cell phone in her hand. The AFE driving her misery

6

caused her to jump and smash her body, allowing the world to mistakenly think she was too delicate, that her pain threshold was too low, that she was not able to stand prenatal pain. In fact, Chinese women are some of the world's most able to tolerate pain. Shawn Ci describes them well: "Chinese women are aware of everything around them; they are the most free, the most self-reliant, the most independent, the most outstanding, the most struggling, the toughest of women. They should be given even more respect and applause than other women."

Since her death, some people have said that Rongrong Ma's husband may have let her bear her pain because he did not want to spend money for a C-section, which is false; ultimately, he was left with unlimited sadness and countless doubts. The negligent on-duty obstetricians and nurses, lacking knowledge and experience, were busy with six deliveries that night and had not anticipated that the hidden and damaging killer would appear. Consequently, the person who was in charge faced suspension and likely felt responsible for the pain and death. The horror of it all is that, similar to after a vicious hurricane, significant loss occurred: deaths of mother and child, pain of family, and damage to reputations of doctors, nurses, and hospital. Like an invisible net, the circumstances became a trap for countless people, exacerbating the destructive turmoil. The doctor bites the bullet, and the innocent must be compensated.

In regard to *a pregnant woman jumping from a window*, I had heard words similar to those thirty-three years ago. In Shenzhen Central Hospital in 1984, I met a pregnant woman who would have had uterine rupture because of cephalopelvic disproportion. I suspected AFE. Caesarean section was implemented in a timely manner, and the patient survived. The situation that occurred that year is still vivid in my mind.

The woman, Xuehua Yang (a pseudonym used for privacy reasons), was at week 40 in her pregnancy and during delivery said that she was in so much pain that she wanted to jump from a window. I gave her psychological counseling and persuaded her to change her mind by saying, "You are going to be a mother. You will persevere and be patient, and you will soon be safe." Fang Fang, a midwife standing next to me, jokingly said to Xuehua Yang, "You are only on the second floor, so if you jumped from here, you would not die." Oh! The inappropriateness of making a remark involving jumping from a window to this pregnant woman got my attention, making me even more alert, and I immediately went to her bedside, reexamined her abdomen, and found that her lower uterine section was tender. Within her abdomen, I could see a pathologically shrinking ringlike area. In order to avoid the threatening uterine rupture, I immediately scheduled the operating room and requested nurses to promptly prepare the patient for C-section by shaving her, anesthetizing her, and disinfecting the surgical site. I washed and sterilized my hands for surgery and then quickly made a conventional cut, a peak-like opening in the abdominal cavity. I cut the uterus open, picked up the baby, cleared the amniotic fluid and the baby's nasal mucus, heard the baby's first wonderful cry, and then cut the umbilical cord and carefully tied off the umbilical cord stump. All the dangers vanished. After twelve hours of close observation, no complications were noted. Disaster was avoided by not waiting for the arrival of the mysterious killing disorder.

It is sad and pitiful that, while I wanted to explore the real causes of a patient's death and make the truth about AFE known to the public so that prevention and treatment could be addressed, other actions were central, and investigation of the situation ended. The hospital is discussing compensation with the family; however, I do not think this is the most meaningful approach. To remedy the situation, timely reflection is necessary. What would be most valuable would be to find the nature of the real culprit, to eliminate its further devastation, to no longer allow pregnant women to face tragedy, to no longer allow AFE to damage and kill mothers and children.

CHAPTER 3
First Encounter with the Killer
初遇杀手

ALL MOTHERS IN THE world, including obstetricians and gynecologists, lack knowledge and understanding of AFE; thus, they lack vigilance and often neglect to confirm its existence. It seems far away but wanders about us every day, depriving the world of numerous mothers, and fetuses that may have continued developing, causing them to succumb to malaise and death. For me, the hidden killer made its appearance in an obstetrics and gynecology department 32 years ago. In August 1978, I was 16 years old and had just been admitted to medical school. On August 13, 1983, at the age of 21, I began practicing as an Ob-Gyn at Shenzhen Central Hospital. I became involved with and fought against AFE at the beginning my lifesaving career, and I was tortured for years because of it. It helped change the direction of my life. I will now describe my experiences in the obstetrics and gynecology department where I practiced 32 years ago on the other side of the Pacific Ocean.

At 5 p.m. on August 13, 1985, on the breezy evening of the mid-autumn festival, my turn on night duty began. I had gone to the obstetrics and gynecology ward after dinner and began my shift on time. During that evening, there were seven maternity cases, one involving a woman 37 weeks pregnant who presented with fetal malformation associated with polyhydramnios and whose fetus was stillborn. The patient, Liping Chen (a pseudonym), was scheduled to have an abortion. Three days earlier, an ultrasound examination showed maternal polyhydramnios, fetal malformations (aphonia), and the absence of a fetal heart beat. Polycythemia vera was suspected. At 11:30 a.m., to induce contractions, oxytocin was administered rhythmically, drop by drop, through the patient's right hand vein. Medical records showed that Liping Chen began to have irregular uterine contractions at 2 p.m., accompanied by a little vaginal bleeding, while blood pressure, pulse, and respiration were normal.

I smiled, said hello to Chen, asked about her diet and emotions, and reminded her to relax and not be too nervous. She was a fair-skinned, beautiful, tall woman. Her beauty was difficult to hide even in her present condition. As the sun shone through the window onto her bulging abdomen, I could clearly see the rectus abdominis pregnancy stretch marks, looking like a gorgeous, glowing colorful sunset. Her husband sat on a stool beside her and peeled an apple with his knife. The pair seemingly made a very loving couple. When I looked at her hill-shaped belly, an uneasy feeling passed through my heart, and I remeasured her abdominal circumference. It was 147 cm (in a full-term pregnant woman, it is normally about 120 cm). I listened to her heart and lungs with a stethoscope and found no abnormalities. I left the ward and took the elevator to the operating room on the 4th floor.

Because of another patient's cephalopelvic disproportion and fetal hypoxia, I needed to perform a C-section immediately. That patient was ready and waiting for me. I followed surgical procedures, skillfully removed a baby girl, and then sutured the uterus and abdominal cavity. Afterward, I removed my heavy surgical gown and then wore only my delivery-room work clothes. I began to easily and carefully write the details in the surgical records. Everything was organized step by step. A rare moment of quiet occurred in the maternity ward, without the fierce battles usual for weekdays. After completing another gynecological examination, I went to recheck the pregnant woman who had too much amniotic fluid. I was uneasy about her mountainous abdomen, concerned about amniotic fluid, and felt a foreboding because of a slightly bloody smell. The delivery room had no air-conditioning or music playing. Instead there were three fans spinning and blowing, and occasionally the groanings of women with uterine contractions were heard.

At 7:30 p.m., Liping Chen began having regular uterine contractions with paroxysmal increase. Her labor had officially started; everything was still calm; no one expected a killer to quietly approach and cause the suffering that was to come! During the paroxysmal uterine contraction, I gave the patient an examination and observed that the cervix had opened three centimeters. With the help of oxytocin, the regular uterine contractions gradually strengthened, each lasting for 60 seconds, intermittently every 5 minutes. Midway through the process, Chen drank a little rice porridge. At 10:13 p.m., I repeated the examination and observed that the cervix was almost completely open (10 centimeters is completely open for all pregnant women at delivery). The second stage of labor had now begun. The midwife immediately moved Liping Chen into the delivery room and transferred her to the birthing bed.

With her legs apart and feet strapped to the stirrups, I taught the patient how to match the rhythm of her uterine contractions to her breath. She grabbed the handles of the birthing bed with both her hands as the uterus contracted and she pushed downward. The cervix had completely opened, but the amniotic membrane had not broken. I used lock forceps to pierce the membrane. The turbid amniotic fluid moved like a rapid stream and immediately shot out of her uterus. Nearly 100 mL spurted toward me, but I escaped from it, thanks to my quick avoidance. Next to me stood Xiaofang, whose face was sprayed with amniotic fluid. Her surgical mask was soaked, and she quickly replaced it with a new one. The color of the fluid was yellow and light green, like the background color in Leonardo da Vinci's *Mona Lisa* (see chapter 18). After the amniotic membrane was punctured, the uterine contractions continued to strengthen paroxysmally, and soon I could see the fetus's black hair.

While the nurse washed off the mother, disinfected the perineum, put a towel in place, and opened a sterile delivery pack, I changed my gloves. The midwife quickly returned to Chen's prenatal bed to protect the perineal raphe during the delivery. When the uterine contractions became very strong, Chen took a deep breath and held it until exhausted. Because of the large size of the fetus, the second labor stage went a little less smoothly. Two sturdy midwives stood beside the patient, whose feet were on the stirrups. One midwife stood on her right side and the other on her left, each holding onto an end of the cloth that would push her abdomen to increase the pressure, pushing the baby downward. At 11:30 p.m., a male child was finally delivered, but he was not breathing; he was stillborn.

The baby's weight was 4 kg, and his length was 50 cm. His abdomen was deformed. The midwife wrapped him up and took him outside the delivery room to allow the patient's husband to see him. Because of an early diagnosis after B-mode ultrasound, the husband was psychologically prepared. When he saw the child's deformity, he looked sad and helpless and silently shook his head. Thirty minutes later, the placenta still had not discharged, so I followed the usual protocol, placing my right hand inside the uterine cavity to perform a placental stripping. Then I sutured the ruptured perineum. At that time, the amount of bleeding was small, about 100 cc in volume.

After the delivery, the silent patient was naturally in pain and in a bad mood. While I sutured her perineum, I tried to console her by saying, "You are young, so don't be too sad. You will be nursed back to health, and you will one day have a healthy child. I'll help you deliver a beautiful baby who will look just like you." She politely replied, "Thank you. You worked hard." Afterward, I stood up and observed her expression. She was breathing smoothly and showed no abnormalities. She was pale, and her face and hair were penetrated with sweat. I asked her how she felt, and she just said, "Thirsty." So I instructed the nurse to give her a glass of water. The midwife indicated that her blood pressure was normal (100/60 mmHg). The delivery room was once again calm, but because I was wearing clothing beneath my surgical gown and had been working so hard, large beads of perspiration had formed on my skin, and I was out of breath.

By the time I had finished with the case, it was the time of evening when the round moon was attended by scattered stars seemingly floating in the sky. The earth was silent, and peace was everywhere. It was already a little past 1:00 a.m. I rinsed off some and hurried back to the doctors' lounge to lie down and try to sleep for a minute or two. Because an emergency could have occurred at any time and one must be prepared to deal with anything, I anticipated a possibly sleepless night. As soon as my head hit the pillow, I entered a deep-sleep state. Who would have expected that the killer, shrouded in darkness, was creeping quietly inside Chen? Sure enough, after I had slept about ten minutes, I heard Xiaofang, the nurse on duty, rapidly, violently knocking at the door. She shouted, "Doctor Lian, Doctor Lian, postpartum hemorrhage at Bed Thirteen!" I awoke suddenly. I jumped up, quickly put on my white coat and high heels, and flew at lightning speed toward the patient. I saw Chen half-lying on the bed with two pillows behind her back, her skin pale, lips cyanotic, facial expression indicating pain, breath short. She was gasping heavily, and her chest was rapidly moving up and down. She could not answer my questions. The thick mat paper under her hips had already been soaked by blood, the volume estimated to have been 400 cc. I measured her blood pressure myself; it had dropped to 50/30 mmHg. Her breath rate was 20/min, and her pulse was 120/min. I listened through a stethoscope and recognized that her lungs were covered with wet rales. The combination of her history of excessive amniotic fluid, fetal malformations, her having had an induced labor and a stillborn infant and the symptoms of dyspnea and postpartum hemorrhage, as well as signs such as having both lungs covered with rales, made for a terrible diagnosis, a most dangerous postpartum complication, which causes greater than 80% mortality. A diagnosis of AFE jumped to my mind. A woman's life was on the line.

The air suddenly seemed solidified, and my blood was like ice. My heart beat rapidly, and my adrenaline soared. I hurriedly instructed the nurse to give the patient oxygen, an intravenous anti-allergy infusion, and medication for pulmonary hypertension, and also to prepare for the blood transfusion and have lab tests performed. Additionally, I reported the situation to the supervising doctor. I saw the situation at that time as calm but changeable, very changeable! I called the internist on duty to ask him to do an emergency consultation. He rushed to do a bedside EKG, which suggested that at the right atrium and right ventricle there was an enlargement accompanied by myocardial strain. I asked the radiologist to come and make a radiograph at her bedside. The report showed a hilar fan-shaped shadow, with a right heart enlargement. A diagnosis of polyhydramniosa, combined with a history of uterine contractions, hyper contractions, dyspnea, cyanosis, shock, signs of major bleeding, and the above test results, indicated more clearly the presence of AFE. The on-duty supervising doctor who heard this news set about to rush the ward guidance work. My heart rose to my throat as the the division of labor cooperated, assuming responsibilities and performing duties methodically, racing against time.

Everyone went all out to perform the rescue work on the patient. The well-trained, skilled nurses were accurate, quick, and agile in implementing the doctors' instructions. Dexamethasone (40 mL) was administered with fluids (following a 20 mg intravenous injection). Low-molecular-weight dextran (1000 mL) was infused intravenously, along with papaverine hydrochloride (60 mg, in basic 10% glucose solution), and 20 mL of atropine (20 mg) was injected intravenously every 20 minutes. Heparin (50 mg) was added to 100 mL of saline and administered within minutes, and subsequently, 500 mL of heparin (50 mg) dissolved in a 5% glucose solution was infused intravenously. With new blood having been transfused into the patient, we were at a critical moment. The hospital's multidisciplinary joint rescue effort was in action, with everyone realizing that time was crucial for the patient's life. Meanwhile, the deadly disorder was still battling to snatch it away. We hoped to overcome death by turning away the danger Chen faced. Her blood pressure had increased, but the bleeding continued. Her blood was not coagulating, and subcutaneous bleeding spots appeared.

The patient's dyspnea symptoms gradually became aggravated, her lip cyanosis increased, and both sides of her nose moved in and out because of hypoxia, causing her to breathe loudly. She was completely unable to answer any questions asked by the doctors or nurses. Her mental state was poor; she was irritable and in a trance-like state. She was extremely agitated and twice ripped out her O_2 tube with her right hand. She pulled out her IV and knocked onto the floor the medicine tray carried by the nurse.

The extremely irritable patient, breathing with great difficulty, was becoming unconscious. She had chills, was vomiting again, and was seemingly tortured by an invisible force, as if she were being swallowed by a serpent, while fighting hard against it. It looked as if a killer was causing her to endure the ultimate torture of death by consuming her, strangling her by the throat, and dragging her into an abyss.

Family members waited anxiously in front of the ward, pacing back and forth, from time to time looking through the window. Blood tests, blood transfusions, infusions, and rescue work continued in an orderly manner. I talked with family members and informed them that the patient was experiencing various syndromes due to prenatal polyhydramnios. Amniotic fluid had entered her heart, lungs, and brain during child-birth, causing her to have heart and lung failure. Her postpartum hemorrhage was caused by the amniotic fluid entering her entire circulatory system, causing disseminated intravascular coagulation (DIC), which is a very violent compli-cation that can occur in obstetrics. Worldwide, the mortality rate from this disease is greater than 80%. The husband's expression was one of extreme pain, but he understood the information, and he shook hands in agreement and then signed the critical-illness form.

That night, all our medical staff was on duty, including the doctors who came to consult and who then returned to assist with rescue efforts. About ten staff members actively worked to save this patient. However, the brutal killer had entered her kidneys, moving her from polyuria to oliguria, anuria, and uremia. Laboratory results for BUN/CO_2 showed they had increased to renal failure levels, and the bleeding continued. We used a lot of hemostatic agents and blood transfusions (total of 2,500 cc), but they were of no use. Soon Chen's organs had gone into the failure stage, and tidal breathing emerged. The patient entered a comatose state. Once again specialists from all disciplines were called for a comprehensive consultation to discuss an optimal treatment plan and to implement it without missing any details. The patient's condition was deteriorating, and the symptoms shifted from previous dyspnea to respiratory failure. We had reached the end of our treatments when we followed the chief physician's advice and transferred her to the intensive care unit (ICU).

Treatment of this patient had begun at around 1:00 a.m. and had continued until about 8:00 a.m. Every second we were in a state of great tension, and I continuously heard a loud drum beating in my heart and felt as if I were walking on an edge. Having worked more than seven hours without stopping, I had no time to drink even a drop of water, let alone go to the toilet. Every cell of my body was in a state of extreme stress, with epinephrine greatly secreted. During that dark night, we worked against the fierce killer, making every effort to save the patient's life, seeking to overcome the disease and bring her back to her previous life. Later, after the patient had been handed over to the ICU's medical specialist for further treatment, I felt some relief. Thank Goodness! Chen finally, luckily, escaped from some of the torture of the long night! However, her vital signs were still at imminent risk. I prayed to God to let her pass through the hell and escape from her robber. I prayed that she would finally overcome AFE and shake off death!

After a night of fighting so hard for the patient on the second floor, my exhaustion, both physical and mental, was extreme. My legs seemed to walk through heaps of cotton, and I experienced loss of balance. At the start of the morning shift, when I left the ward, my body so weary, I saw the equally tired husband of the overwhelmed patient, who stood stooped against the promenade, gazing into the sky as if praying. Hearing footsteps, he turned to look at me. I noticed his helpless, painful, and desperate expression. I think he saw the same expression on my face. Neither of us said hello or spoke. I recognized a man who was about to lose his wife, and I understood his miserable heart. Though a doctor, I felt inferior to him in his pain. His situation was the more heartbreaking. But we at the hospital were all in a similar sad mood. Although I tried my best, I felt guilty about not being able to avert her death. The next day at 4:17 p.m., Liping Chen died of systemic failure caused by the AFE. The pathology report also confirmed the clinical diagnosis of amniotic fluid embolism. Now more than 32 years have passed, yet I can still remember the desperate look of the patient's husband. If one becomes aware of complications, is it not better to choose C-section as the delivery method? Will family members in the future agree to surgery for delivering a stillborn infant? Might AFE occur during C-section? During the delivery of a stillborn infant, might two robust midwives

holding a cloth over an abdomen cause or aggra-
vate AFE? Is the cause a single factor or a combination of factors? What is the main reason for
AFE? How can this tragedy be avoided? What is
the best protocol for saving a patient? How can
early detection and timely diagnosis be achieved?
What medicine is the most effective? What dose is
the most appropriate? Which parts of diagnosis
and treatment may cause problems? I have been
searching for answers.

CHAPTER 4
Why Did She Hit the Doctor?
相煎何急

AFTER LEARNING OF A suicide by jumping in Yulin, Shaanxi Province, China, I stayed awake all night. The next morning, I sat on a wide balcony, listening to melodious music while gazing at my backyard that was drenched in the Florida sun and noticing the sparkling of a crystal blue lake in the autumn wind. In the swimming pool, a Feng Shui ball was lit up by the sun. Also, golden turtle eggs were illuminated on the surface. On the ground was an ancient tree uprooted by a hurricane. In my concern about the suicide, I continued to use my cell phone to search for more reports and any progress made on the case. I read each word in a serious manner, looking for anything that might be helpful, thinking and hoping that I might find clues by reading between the lines.

A tragic scene caused by the hidden, strange, deadly disorder of thirty years ago had emerged again on August 31, 1987. Coincidentally, it was the same day and same month that the other suicide by jumping occurred. I had been promoted by the Shenzhen Municipal Central Hospital, the South's oldest and number one hospital, the Zhongshan Medical University's First Affiliated Hospital, to practice one year of obstetrics and gynecology. At about 10:00 a.m., I walked from the department of medicine to the outpatient department. The sun was bright, the weather was warm and fine, and the vibrant scarlet kapok tree flowers were blooming and swaying in the wind. Accompanied by the delightful fragrance of the osmanthus flowers everywhere in the gardens of the medical school, the beautiful songs of the birds could be heard.

Beautiful, young, and full of vitality, I, wearing a white coat and with shiny, thick black hair covering my shoulders, walked on in my high heels, enjoying the pleasant view of the hospital gardens, humming a little Hakka song, and feeling great pleasure. I headed down the slope, and Dr. Tan, who was the Ob-Gyn professor, walked up toward me, her delicate white skin, medium stature, and flowing curves noticeable. Dressed as she was in her white coat, she looked full of spirit, with the dignity of a medical professor. We smiled and cordially greeted each other. Suddenly, a bicycle appeared at my right-hand side, ridden by a middle-aged woman. With lightning speed, she jumped off and pounced like a lioness at Dr. Tan. The woman's fist beat into her body, wounding her. I was shocked and instinctively rushed forward and with both hands held the attacker's waist tightly. She struggled hard but was not able to break free. Then she mercilessly pulled up her right heel and stamped hard into my right thigh, causing pain to burst through my body.

I endured the pain while tightly holding onto the woman, but she struggled hard, cursing, and rushed forward toward Dr. Tan, as if Dr. Tan were a culprit. In her deep hatred, she wanted to tear her down, as if "taking revenge against her father." Fortunately, hospital security hurried over in time to quell further development of the incident by pulling the woman away, forcing her to hold back her bitter anger at Dr. Tan's departure, and seemingly causing her whole body to react in mournful pain. I helped Dr. Tan walk to the doctor's clinic. The nurse there measured her blood pressure, which had risen to 230/100 mmHg, and her heart rate, which was 120/min. Dr. Tan looked very pale, her whole body was shaking, and her eyes were filled with tears of humiliation that then burst like a waterfall onto her whole face. This scene made me sad and distressed, and so far it has been unforgettable!

It was puzzling to me that the hospital did not deal with this woman who had attacked a doctor in public. The next morning, on the second floor, in the baby room, I saw her again. The nurses were feeding milk to an approximately two-month-old boy. I had no idea why such a big boy was in the room. I rushed forward and with my right hand pointed indignantly at the woman said, "Hey! Why did you beat up on Dr. Tan yesterday, fighting her to the death?!" She put her hands on her waist and answered me, saying, "You are a new doctor—you don't know what happened!" Then a nurse came over, pulled me aside, and quietly told me that the little boy was the woman's grandson. Two months previously, her daughter unfortunately died from AFE in our hospital. She blamed the doctors and nurses, and whenever she saw those who had been on duty during the delivery, she rushed over and began behaving crazy, hitting them hard. At the same time, her son-in-law kept writing letters to the Yangcheng Evening News and the Nanfang Daily to complain about the hospital.

On that particular case, nurses participated in the rescue effort for more than ten consecutive hours, and more than 3,000 cc of blood was transfused to the patient. The staff had done its best. It turned out that Dr. Tan was one of two doctors who had participated in the rescue effort. Oh!—I soon realized why a doctor of obstetrics and gynecology must always look around before leaving work and should check as to whether any suspicious persons are outside the delivery room before daring to go home, especially taking note of any odd intuition. Now I understood. A heart cannot help but break, and tears cannot help but flow under such circumstances. I deeply sympathized with the grandmother who lost her daughter and had to raise her grandson alone. I deeply sympathized with the orphan who lost his mother at birth. I deeply sympathized with the doctors involved in the rescue effort and with my professors, and I sympathized even more deeply because the strange, vicious killer that I hated was the cause!

The miserable, hateful grandmother—at middle age, at a time in her life that should have been the best—could have lived in wonderful retirement, enjoying the happiness of three gen-erations of her family, but instead she had en-countered this tragedy. The little grandson, who normally would have been welcomed into her life, became a representation of her grief after her only daughter's life had been stolen. A fateful storm had suddenly carried her off into a void. As the saying goes, "The hearts of a mother and daughter are connected to each other." The mother lost her daughter for no good reason. Her son-in-law in his pain could not take care of a child. How could an old woman in her roles of both grandmother and mother not help feeling extreme anger? And who could soothe her lonely, painful soul? She was stimulated to vent that pain and anger toward the medical staff. After a lapse of thirty years, I still remember it vividly. Although so many years have passed, the wound still aches. The torture inflicted by AFE, whether on minds, bodies, or spirits, become hard-to-remove scars. Although I did not participate in that particular event, because of my participation in other rescue cases involving bleeding conditions, I realize that all doctors, including primary care physicians, residents, professors, and visiting doctors, along with nurses, work together to make every effort, day and night, to rescue their patients, using the best medicines and medical technology. Many rescue efforts are successful, but rescue from AFE is obviously rare, with its 80% fatality rate worldwide (some even report a mortality rate of over 90%). My colleagues, after doing everything in their power to reverse AFE, have also suffered, some having left the hospital, and some having experienced violence from the families. I still feel the pain of their experiences, which is why I write about this subject. Injustice owes them a debt because they were not the killer, rather it was AFE! This embolism is our common enemy, and I would like to say to the mother who lost her daughter, "Those who attempted to save your daughter—the doctors and nurses—are also parents, and they have the hearts of parents, so do not think of them as your foes. Because of your daughter's death, they too have suffered!"

Also, I pray for the child who lost his mother. Perhaps he lives a happy life and may soon marry. Medical doctors have hearts, and they would hope his relatives would not attribute his mother's death to them or to nurses but instead to the embolism. Zhongshan Medical College doctors have the best technology and medical skills. I interviewed a lot of rescue staff who were present at the time; they do their best. The death rate in the US is also greater than 80%. I regret this situation, because healing the sick is a doctor's sacred duty. If we could find better treatments for saving lives, we would even sacrifice ourselves to a hungry tiger, as Sakyamuni Buddha did. Yes, we would be willing to do so!

CHAPTER 5
Pitiful Xiaoqiang
小强可怜

I REMEMBER THAT IN my youth my grandfather had a patient who was born less than 24 hours before his 20-year-old mother died. Locals called him the white tiger reincarnated. They said his mother died because she was pregnant with this ghost; they said Xiaoqiang was his mother's killer. In fact, his mother most likely died of AFE. My grandfather once mentioned to me that her body was "dirty" from the amniotic fluid that invaded her body and caused bleeding and death. Back then the concept was unscientific and super-stitious. Whereas now we have an understanding of this disorder, at that time it was impossible to see the dangerous postnatal complications from a scientific, rational point of view. Thus, the death was attributed to the infant, and the unfortunate child was regarded as an ominous symbol.

That poor child, Xiaoqiang, was said to have been lying in wait before being born into this world. Often other children verbally abused and assaulted him. He silently endured the prejudices of and the injuries by people around him. He was small but strong as a six-year old. In height and weight he was only as large as a four-year-old. His usually silent, handsome little face always expressed melancholy, and his sad eyes often stared blankly at the sky. When gazing at a night sky filled with stars, especially when staring at the desolate autumn moon, he may have been seeing heaven in the distance and missing his mother. He was strong, ragged, unpretentious, and often cold and hungry. My good grandparents and mother, who were sympathetic to poor Xiaoqiang, often gave him special care such as free treatment and food. Later, Xiaoqiang's father remarried. The stepmother was unkind to him, often scolding him, giving him only sweet potatoes and porridge to eat, and only at the New Year giving him a little meat, and rarely fresh fish. When Xiaoqiang was about seven years old, he wanted to help with the housework. At eight years old, he helped with the ducks and chickens. Even on windy and rainy days, Xiaoqiang had to herd the ducks outside. Whenever a storm came, he used bamboo poles to catch them, and then, facing the thunderstorm, he waved to the heavens and cried to the sky, as if to say it was unfortunate and unfair that it had become dark this early. Because of his birth defects, coupled with his malnutrition, and because he suffered from cervical lymph node tuberculosis, he often had a low-grade fever by the afternoon. He had a large mass in his neck. At that time, his father brought him to see my grandfather for medical treatment. He looked very handsome, with his big, exceptionally bright eyes. He walked a kilometer each day to his school, in the hot summer and the freezing winter, and that helped to make him self-reliant and self-confident. In academic achievement he was always among the best in his class.

He wrote an essay titled *Mother, I Miss You. Mother, Where Are You?* Between the lines his words revealed deep-felt thoughts of the mother he never knew and the sadness and sorrow of being an orphan. "Mother, where have you been? Please come home quickly . . . ," he implored. His essay caused many people to be moved to tears for his sorrow. His mother's death and his resultant suffering touched me so much that I was determined to become an Ob-Gyn and save women like his mother so that children like him would not become orphans.

CHAPTER 6
Away From My Hometown
远走他乡

FROM THE TIME I was young, I was determined to become a good doctor. With Dr. Qiaoya Lin as an example, I hoped to become an excellent Ob-Gyn. During my wonderful youthful life, in medical school, I always studied hard, not even going out to watch movies, to be entertained, or to date. I also rejected a lot of good suitors. My whole mind and body were focused on future patients and my sacred cause. My first encounter with AFE not only took away a patient's life and put her family and me in pain. It also changed my life's path.

I had a high school classmate, who, like me, was a straight-A student at the top of the class, and who said he loved me with the purest and sincerest love. He was good, dignified, gentle, diligent, and motivated. He did not talk a lot, which made just the right yin and yang balance with my extroverted personality. When he was in college, he kept writing to me and expressed his intention. Both sets of parents expressed their satisfaction with the match, believing that we made a good couple. But my medical school education was intense, and I only wanted to concentrate on studying and becoming a good doctor. I placed my pursuit of this cause even higher than my emotional needs and family demands, with an idea that love was not an option and was to be avoided. So I rejected his marriage proposal. But our two hearts were interlinked. I still had him, and he still had me. I would have been a happy bride and wife. However, ever since I encountered AFE, the pressure I felt was so great that the patient's pale and gasping face often swayed in front of me, as if to say that the demon that had killed her was still at large.

I often felt anxious, as if in the midst of a horror, wandering in darkness, my heart full of sadness, while continuing to work hard. I felt as if my soul had been pumped away. I was close to the brink of collapse. The killer had entered my personal life, and I suffered from the aftermath. Often, though sleeping little, I dreamed of being in the depths of a jungle where I saw animals and elves joyfully dancing and then suddenly smirking with a *Mona Lisa*-like expression on a killer's face. In my dream, the patient Chen was in a monster's hands, and she cried out for help, while I tried hard to pull her by the hand. In a colorful, alien world, the *Transformer*-like killer had strength greater than mine and pulled at Chen's throat, pulling her to an unknown place, leaving only a red mess in the white snow covering the ground, which became a beach of uncoagulated, flowing blood, snow white yet blood red.

This dream appeared more than once in the dead of night, and sometimes it became even more cruel and appalling, with Chen being bitten tightly by a bloodthirsty wolf, its wrecked, sharp teeth spurting blood. Although I held onto the wolf with one hand, I could not find a place on its head where I could beat it with all the bitterness I felt. It was neverthless able to slaughter my patient. The two sides fought—yet I was unable to stop the ripping force. I was haunted by lost opportunities and doubts, and I often awoke sweating after such a nightmare. Then I would burst into tears, not able to stop crying. I had been a witness to a demon's existence, and it was still at large with impunity. This cast a long psychological shadow. I was deeply distressed, worried, troubled. And so was each doctor in the department of medicine who was in charge of the 24 beds, who saw more than 60 patients a day, and who had heavy work pressures and respon-sibilies, along with complex human experiences and personal relationships. I walked on the edge of the edge, often in fear and confusion.

No one gave me any help at this time when I most needed to have my broken heart comforted. With no psychological counseling, my jumpy nerves silently endured. I then ran into the arms of another surgeon to find relief from my empti-ness and mental stress. I married him in a hurry, having formally rejected the man who loved me three times. He heard that I had married, and, helpless to remedy the situation, he could only marry someone else. We might have had a life-time of love, growing prosperous together, having children and grandchildren. But I believed in myself, that I would be a most virtuous wife, and that my new husband and I would fly away to-gether. I had hoped my marriage would give me a safe haven and would eliminate the killer's shadow, but it was not meant to be. I had run to a pious hypocrite. The marriage was intolerable, so I bared myself in court to obtain a divorce. The combination of the mysterious killer, the unfortu-nate marriage, and the divorce caused me to re-solve to leave the Shenzhen Central Hospital Office and to say farewell to obstetrics and gyne-cology.

Bitao Lian

In January 1990, carrying two heavy suit-cases loaded with medical books, I crossed the Lo Wu Bridge, flew over the South Pacific Ocean to Sydney, Australia, and then integrated myself in-to study at my own expense. I had a bitter, lone-ly heart, having bid farewell to family, friends, patients, hospital colleagues, and to a life in ob-stetrics and gynecology, and found myself faraway from home. Originally I had wanted to go abroad to learn advanced technology and do research on AFE. I wanted to grasp and catch the killing, bloodthirsty devil—and find his secret weapon. I wanted to capture this ghost, and I felt I was on the clock. I planned to eventually return to the Shenzhen Municipal Central Hospital to continue my career as an Ob-Gyn, but instead I began traveling down a road of no return.

In Australia, gazing at the blue water below the Sydney Opera House and the Sydney Harbour Bridge, I often thought about amniotic fluid and became fretful and confused, mindful of the horror of embolism. While studying there, I was also a practitioner at Sydney's Chinese Herbs Medical Center in Chinatown. In the absence of hospital obstetrics and gynecology, I had no chance of exposure to the killer, but from hearsay I learned of a 30-year-old Chinese woman who had died of postpartum hemorrhage. The cause was said to have been AFE. Because it was not firshand information, I could not give an opinion. In the fall of 1992, I moved from Sydney and its beautiful, pleasant climate, leaving my classmates, friends, and patients, and emigrated to Florida. When I first arrived, I was very unfamiliar with the way of life there. But I have many skills and so was able to quickly adapt to the environment and pass the Florida Acupuncturist Licensing Examination.

However, late at night, often looking up at the moonlight before falling asleep, I missed my family and friends. I missed the Shenzhen Municipal Central Hospital obstetrics and gynecology department and often dreamed of patients in surgery and of anxiously asking the nurse beside me to hand me scissors and forceps. I dreamed of the rupture during labor and of clear or cloudy amniotic fluid. Often in my dreams, I rushed forward in battle, even able to vaguely see the smile on the killer's devilish face before waking up! Although I lived on the the other side of the world, I found the same killer. Meanwhile, I constantly looked for information about AFE in foreign literature and domestic news.

CHAPTER 7
A Serial Killer
连环杀手

ON SEPTEMBER 20, 1994, on the day of China's traditional mid-autumn festival, I had just arrived from the US to visit my family in Shenzhen, Guangdong Province. On that day, my grandfather, grandmother, father, mother, and I were busy buying moon cakes, grapefruit, and peanuts for the festival. Suddenly, at about 10 a.m., gunfire was heard on a Hong Kong television-news program. Mingjian Tian, age 30, Lieutenant Commander of the Twelfth Division of the Third Command Division of the Beijing People's Liberation Army, stationed in Tongxian County, suddenly shot and killed four commissar group officers, who were his fellow officers. Carrying a gun, he then hijacked a jeep and ordered the driver to speed toward Tiananmen Square. Running a red light, the driver crashed into a tree, where Mingjian Tian was eventually shot dead.

Both the military and police had rushed to the scene to stop Mingjian Tian, and a fierce gun battle ensued. The two sides violently exchanged fire on both sides of the city road, with as many as seven armed police officers reportedly killed in the crossfire. During the battle, a 44-seat bus entered the area, where the driver stopped, panic-stricken, and significant casualty of the passengers resulted. In addition, a number of civilians who were passing by were killed or wounded. The victims included Yusuf Mohammad Pishjoneri, the government's Iranian Embassy secretary, who was inside a car along with his nine-year-old son. Two children were injured. The rogue officer who had tried to escape was nearly exhausted and was shot in the face by a military unit that had rushed in. According to Beijing Forensic Laboratory Identification Center statistics, a total of 75 people died or were wounded because of the vicious incident.

On that day, the Xinhua News Agency published an article of more than a hundred words in the Beijing Evening News. Someone had once said, "People buy newspapers." Details of the sensational story were in high demand, making appropriate the Chinese expression "Paper is expensive in Luoyang." What had happened to turn Mingjian Tian, who should have been loyal to his fellow officers, into a murderer? While everyone was deeply upset about the innocent civilians' deaths, they especially wanted to determine the root of the crime. Foreign sources reported that the incident had been caused by the Chinese government's family planning policy. The murderer's wife, who had declined to have an abortion, was said to have been responsible for the death of both herself and their child. The army's investigative team reported that Mingjian Tian was consistently outdone by his soldiers, not only at war but also by the presents they gave to regiment leaders, which were bribes for promotions. Whenever soldiers requested leave to visit their families out of town, Mingjian Tian opposed them and then met with military officers to discuss dismissing them. When higher authorities learned of these behaviors, they decided to reorganize. In the meantime, a trustee who had received a gift from Mingjian Tian had returned his gift. It was speculated that Mingjian Tian, thinking he had no chance for promotion, decided to retaliate.

The incident alarmed the Central Military Commission Chairman, Zemin Jiang. He too wondered what had motivated the man to turn to mad retaliation and destruction. My answer is AFE. Mingjian Tian, who had a daughter and also wanted a son, was struggling because his wife, seven months pregnant, was not allowed by the government to have a second child. She was forced by the local government to have an abortion. The infant died during forced labor induction, and she subsequently died because of bleeding. At her first delivery, both she and her child had been healthy.

In obstetrics and gynecology, it is well known that women who have given birth at least once are physically different from first-time pregnant women (primipara). A woman who has delivered at least one child is like a tested, tempered veteran on a battlefield. For such a woman, the first and second labor stages are significantly shortened, and other factors, such as heart disease, hyperthyroidism, and hypertension, are of less concern. Women are said to become more powerful through the delivery process. In patients' records, obstetricians write "P: __" and "G: __" to indicate the number of pregnancies and childbirths. If a pregnancy is at the stage between 16 and 38 weeks, termination can be accomplished by injecting 5 cc of Rivanol into the amniotic fluid in the uterus and then waiting 24 to 48 hours. The patient will automatically have contractions and bleeding and will then discharge the stillborn or, sometimes, live infant. For Mingjian Tian's wife, there was no suspicion of dysfunction. Generally, obstetric veterans have normal pelvic physiology. After a first child has been born, the second infant is usually safe.

Labor induction has led to a large number of bleeding cases in which death has occurred within 24 hours. The women become irritable because they are in pain and have poor blood circulation, strong contractions, and charged emotions due to the information conducted through nerves and meridians. When emotions are especially high, the conductive nerves can be destroyed, causing blockages and damage. Meridian disorders and AFE can occur under these conditions. In a majority of such cases, the possibility of AFE is high. Mingjian Tian's wife had a greater chance of having AFE because of her psychological state, caused by her anger and other emotions, which resulted from the government taking away her baby. According to statistics, when labor occurs by forced induction, the incidence of death from AFE is 0.86%.

Mingjian Tian's wife and infant were likely destroyed by AFE. She may have lost her mind in her pain and despair. At the same time, Mingjian Tian's ideals, career, and life were destroyed. He was a man who had made his own career. Military personnel, learning of his wife's and son's deaths, believed Mingjian Tian had murdered as a reaction to those tragedies. In the investigative report, it was impossible to connect his violence to the soldiers' bribes or other such matters, if those were even mentioned. One day prior to the incident, Mingjian Tian told a fellow soldier that he should make sure to lie down at his command, as he did not want to hurt his "brother." He was a professional soldier with rural roots, and he longed to have a son who would become a sup-port in his life. The loss of his wife and son, to-gether with his disappointment in the military, may have caused him to lose control and become violent. Unfortunately, no one paid attention to his need for psychological counseling.

With his hopes and dreams ruined, his grud-ges, anger, and pain turned into violent terror, and he became a crazed killer who committed a heinous crime. Thus, Mingjian Tian was likely also an AFE victim, although many external factors were certainly present. For his wife and son, induced abortion was the main, internalized cause. External causes can intensify internal factors. Mingjian Tian believed the government's one-child policy was to blame, and this resulted in mad retaliation toward society. With gun in hand, he stormed the troops—with an amniotic fluid embolus as the impetus! Amniotic fluid embolism was the unknown momentum that mobilized the devil hidden in his heart. He was not able to defeat that devil.

After causing 75 innocent people to be in-jured or killed, Mingjian Tian died from a gunshot wound. Was AFE really to blame? Many people have warned me against writing about these painful memories. But I want to share my know-ledge because the people in the army were my brothers, "my hands and my feet," as we say in China. This incident was not about killing enemies on the battlefield or protecting the peace. Inno-cents were killed, and what a painful human trag-edy it was! The real killer, which caused a series of bloody events, was an amniotic fluid embolus.

Most servicemen's wives are of childbearing age, and they live separately from their husbands most of the time. During childbirth, complications can occur that are easily misunderstood and mis-represented. At the same time, military person-nel, made of flesh and blood, are armed with weapons, and they know that one incident can begin a chain reaction that can end in many deaths. Then why would a military expert cause bloodshed off the battlefield, turning himself into a murderer of innocent people? Is the root cause not worth pondering? The US is paying more attention than China in this regard. Even when landlords attempt to evict tenants, they must first show that those tenants never served in the mili-tary. Similarly, for doctors, it can be quite neces-sary to actively appease anxious, nervous, and fearful patients, especially well-trained former soldiers. The strange, deadly disorder AFE is a sharpshooter of sorts, a mighty force to be reck-oned with, which should arouse the vigilance needed to defuse the fire aimed at the innocent. It is gratifying to note that a new policy allowing parents to have a second child is now in effect in China. A severe one-child policy is hard to imag-ine if one has not lived with it.

I will now describe another sad and unforget-table scene. That incident occurred during the second half of 1982, when I was a student resi-dent in obstetrics and gynecology at Guangzhou Women and Baby Hospital. One day I was as-signed to an abortion room. I wore a white lab coat and a mask, and I stood quietly and respect-fully at the left rear of an operating table. With concentrated eyes, I watched a gynecologist per-form an abortion on a patient. I saw her expand the patient's cervix, insert a tube, and press the foot pedal of an evacuating instrument. With her right hand she held onto a tube, and soon the fetal villi tissue passed out through it into a glass container on the floor. The doctor was highly skilled, and the abortion took about fifteen minutes to complete. She then used a small, metal, fork-like instrument to pick up a round, metal intrauterine device (IUD) and insert it into the patient's uterine cavity. Suddenly, in a tearful voice, the patient said, "Doctor, I'm not married yet." At that moment, a second doctor who stood at the side said in a firm, unrelenting voice, "This is the superior's order." The patient cried painfully and was finally able to leave the operating room, while the two doctors continued to discuss the situation. "Next time, put the IUD into the patient without letting her see it. Your hand was positioned too high, and she was able to see the device," the doctor said.

In the past, with China's one-child family policy, an Ob-Gyn was the implementer of that policy. The political system stipulated that, after a husband and wife's first child was born, an IUD must be inserted into the wife. Also, a couple must first have a permit to have a child after marriage. In one particular case, a married woman surnamed Huang, who was more than two months pregnant and did not have a permit document, was told to have an abortion. Subsequently, she attempted suicide by swallowing 100 sleeping pills and was later found and sent to our hospital emergency room. Gastric lavage was performed using potassium permanganate. Also, sodium sulfate catharsis was done and other measures were taken during the rescue effort. The patient was awoken and transferred to my ward, where my supervisor performed an abortion. I can still remember her closed eyes and pale look.

I also remember a morning in 1985, at the obstetrics and gynecology department of Shenzhen Central Hospital, when a patient who had been pregnant with a second child for more than three months was admitted. In accordance with the one-child policy, she was scheduled to have an abortion at Fu Yong Town Hospital in Bao'an County, where a long plastic catheter was inserted into her uterine cavity. However, she sneaked out of the hospital and ten days later was arrested by law enforcement officers and then sent to our hospital. She was assigned to one of my beds to undergo a labor induction procedure. When I performed a vaginal wash and took out the plastic tube, a bad smell burst out. The treatment room was soon filled with the dis- gusting, vomit-inducing smell of decay. I used the phrase *stinks to high heaven* (臭气熏天)*!* when I described it in her medical records. The good news is that I was fully aware of the importance of using strong antibiotics in sufficient amounts to fight infection, pre- and post-operatively, and I made sure the area was appropriately disinfected during labor induction. The patient was kept safe and finally discharged.

As previously mentioned, policy stipulated that an IUD be inserted after childbirth. If a gov- ernment employee was discovered to have had a second child, that person would have been ex- pelled from both the communist party and any public job held. If a second child was born to rural parents, ligation sterilization would have been required. I performed ligation sterilization on a patient after her second childbirth. She asked to breastfeed her son before the surgery, which I allowed. The boy at her chest was so lovely that I pinched his nose and cheeks, playing with him. The woman explained to me how she had gotten scars on her right forehead. Three months earlier, late at night, her husband flew home to hide in the countryside from family planning office staff. Because of the meandering mountain road and his driving while in a panic-stricken state, their car rolled over and crashed into the woods. Her husband was severely wounded and was still bed-ridden. Her forehead had been cut by broken glass, requiring her to get a dozen stitches. Fortunately, the fetus was not harmed. They were forced to pay a fine of 20,000 Yuan and have the tubal ligation sterilization performed immediately after the childbirth. There is much that can be said about family planning in its relationship to pregnancy complications and AFE, but I have no more to say about it here. The situation changed somewhat in 2015 with a new policy that allows a married couple to have "two full children." Congratulations are in order.

CHAPTER 8
American Women
美国产妇

IN 1993, AFTER OBTAINING my acupuncture license, I opened the Oriental Healing Center in Gainesville, Florida, which has a solid theoretical foundation built on traditional Chinese medicine and western medicine. I use my clinical experience of more than a dozen years, and I work hard and continue to study. It is both a wonderful way to practice medicine and a better tradition in medicine. Besides, I have no fear of illness or the outstanding Chinese tradition. My medical skills are excellent, and I quickly get rid of diseases, heal a lot of difficult illnesses, and earn my patients' respect and trust.

Last month a patient called Maggie (a pseudonym) chatted with me as I adjusted an acupuncture needle during back-pain treatment. On the previous day, in the local teaching hospital, her husband's colleague had suddenly died after having given birth. She was Caucasian, only 26 years old, very healthy, and optimistic. When my patient's husband called her at the hospital to congratulate her, her husband answered the phone and said, "Baby is good, but Mom is dead."

She said to me, "I know you were an experienced Ob-Gyn in China. Please, can you tell me what might have caused this woman to die? How could such a healthy young person have suddenly died after having a smooth childbirth? It was a natural birth, and the labor process went well. Why would she have died within 24 hours? The hospital is first rate. Its brain research center is the largest center invested in by the U.S. Army. The hospital has medical experts and the world's best equipment and medicines." While listening to my patient, my heart tightened, and I asked her if the woman had had certain symptoms before her death, such as contractions, dyspnea, and postpartum hemorrhage. She did not know the exact situation. I began to think of AFE, the strange disorder. My knowledge and understanding, my intuition, told me that the mother had died of this postpartum complication. I then said to my patient that, based on my experience in China, her husband's colleague had died of AFE. She listened, a bit noncommittal. I read the doubt on her face. "Although I admit that you are brilliant, you did not see the patient or treat her, so how can you know that? How can you say she died of that?" she asked. At eleven-thirty that night, I received an email from Maggie. I quickly read, "Dear Doctor, you really are a wise woman. I asked my husband about his colleague's death. The hospital report showed that the cause of her death was the embolism that you mentioned at the clinic today. That is really amazing, godlike! I really admire you!"

I immediately replied to her to say that I was not like God, but that I had met with this weird killer thirty-two years ago. Mothers' lives, obstetrics, gynecology, blood, and tears are what I can understand. I have been entangled with this devil all these years, and I use what I learned to try to expose the hidden disorder that causes pain in healthy bodies and madness in innocent minds by flowing through the bloodstream. I hope to arouse the attention of the entire world. Improvement in

China's standard of living and the decrease in maternal and infant mortality have become important to national policy.

As a leading cause of maternal death, AFE reportedly occurred in 1 in 40,000 North American deliveries in 2016, and in 1 in 53,800 European deliveries the same year. A medical report by the AFE Foundation was reviewed by Debra Sullivan, PhD, MSN, RN, CNE, COI, on October 7, 2016. Amanda Delgago, of the AFE Foundation, wrote that the disorder is rare. Although estimates of incidence numbers vary, it is a leading cause of death that occurs during labor or shortly after birth. The countries in which AFE is a high-ranking cause of death include Australia, France, Japan, and Poland. Statistics on AFE were reported by the US National Institutes of Health in 2009, when only 9 cases of AFE occurred in the US.

Sometime after Maggie told me about her husband's colleague, I asked her to get more information about the situation. "Had her husband filed a lawsuit against the hospital?" I wanted to know. The answer was no. The family had not taken any steps that would have distressed the doctors and nurses there, much less been violent toward them. The husband had asked a lawyer whether there was a possible case. After searching for cases of AFE, the lawyer told him that neither he nor the family would receive any compensation if the hospital were sued. The hospital had informed them during the rescue effort that a fierce postpartum syndrome, AFE, was present. Also, the hospital Ob-Gyns and nurses had given a timely diagnosis and proper treatment and informed them that the world mortality rate is greater than 80%. Family members signed a critical-illness form, and counsel did not consider them to have a strong case. Additionally, the hospital performed an autopsy after the family members agreed to it. Pathologists found tangible fetal material in the amniotic fluid, lungs, and peripheral blood of the mother. Even if the family had engaged the nation's best lawyers, a good chance of winning a case was highly unlikely.

CHAPTER 9
Many Incidences in the Fall
多故之秋

AS WE QUIETLY ENJOY the poetic beauty of our autumn scenery, westerly winds blow across our yards, making it difficult for any butterflies that may be passing through. I have been doing research on AFE and find that more than 90% of the time it occurs in July, August, September, or October. Those are also the months of hurricane season, going along with the old phrase *troubled times in the fall* (多事之秋). Modern medicine has shown that in the human brain the pineal gland secretes melatonin, a hormone that induces people to fall asleep and also causes seasonal depression. Kelly Rohan, a professor of psychology at the University of Vermont, points out that melatonin levels usually increase during the night, causing sleep, and diminish in the morning, causing people to wake up. With autumn and winter daylight hours shortened, this physiological process may be out of balance, plunging some people into a whole season of depression. Melatonin will inhibit the body's thyroid hormone, adrenaline, and other hormones, so that their concentrations are relatively reduced. Thyroxine and epinephrine are the hormones that stimulate the cells to work. After a relative decrease in these hormones, people often feel depressed, perhaps emotional. Melatonin secretion is regulated by the sun; thus, during autumn, when the weather is relatively cooler and dimmer, sunlight exposure is decreased, melatonin secretion is increased, and depression incidence is increased.

As temperatures drop even more, the human body increases oxygen consumption to maintain normal body temperature, vasoconstriction, blood pressure, and heart rate, and the heart's burden increases accordingly. In addition, changes in temperature can exhaust the body's immune cells, decreasing immunity, possibly leading to respiratory infections, affecting lung ventilation function, and increasing relative myocardial hypoxia. Also, cold weather can make blood flow more slowly because of increasing blood viscosity, thus affecting coronary blood supply and increasing thrombus formation. In one of his poems, Li He of the Tang Dynasty declares, "At the place where Nu Wa melted down stones to repair the sky, rock shattered, heaven shook, and autumn rain fell." He reminisces about the unusual autumn, characterizing this time of the year. Autumn can be a worrisome season, especially to a pregnant woman whose delivery date is during that time. If that is the case, medical staff must be more vigilant in preparing for AFE. Because the temperature difference between day and night is larger during autumn, pregnant women are encouraged to drink a chestnut-ginger-jujube drink, which has a warming effect. It is prepared by combining 100 grams of chestnut, 8 grams of jujube, and 15 grams of ginger and should be drunk two to three times a week.

Summer goes, and the cool autumn comes. In the doctrine of the five elements of Chinese medicine, the five internal organs are connected with the four seasons of nature. The lung is mainly connected to autumn; the lung and autumn belong to the same five elements of gold, and they communicate with each other. Autumn is cool and dry, and the lungs are like filters. Lungs like moisture rather than dryness. So it is easy to see that dry-lung syndrome can occur in autumn, causing a clinical cough without sputum, a dry mouth and nose, and cracking, dry skin. How can one get rid of dry lung? Chinese medicine has good methods to do so. Chinese yin herbs have a moisturizing and heating effect. Commonly used Chinese herbs are Ophiopogon, Lily, North Adenophora, and Polygonatum. Methods for increasing lung function during autumn include the following treatment for pregnant women, especially those with chronic bronchitis: blowing up balloons, 30 per day, to help maintain the elasticity of lung cells and bronchi and increase their vital capacities. Pregnant women should take many preventive measures to enhance their physical fitness.

CHAPTER 10
Know Your Enemy
知己知彼

SUN TZU SAID, "KNOW your enemy." In the US, I conducted a thousand surveys on AFE awareness. The people surveyed were patients from my clinic, students from medical schools, WeChat groups, and even people I met on the street. The participants were predominantly American (70%) and Chinese (20%); the rest (10%) were Korean, Japanese, and German, and even included one Haitian (who was an acupuncture student). The survey indicated that only 12% of the surveyed population had a preliminary understanding of AFE. Only the US lawyer Jose I. Moreno had a more profound understanding of the disease. He had done research on it because he was hired by the husband of a woman who had died of AFE during childbirth.

Amniotic fluid, which is present in the amniotic cavity of the uterus during pregnancy, contains the source of life, and I am one of a very few people in the world who have witnessed that life in its first, most primitive stage. That event occurred on New Year's Day in 1983. My patient had been pregnant for 43 days and unfortunately had an ectopic pregnancy. When I opened her abdominal cavity, I saw a beautiful, unforgettable scene: on the left side of the fallopian tube ampulla was a crystal ball–like human embryo, approximately 0.8 cm in size, with a green bean–sized heart regularly beating, surrounded by clear amniotic fluid. I felt as if I were viewing a fairyland.

Amniotic fluid is an indispensable component of the fetus's life throughout pregnancy. During different stages of development, the sources of amniotic fluid vary. In the first trimester of pregnancy, this fluid mainly comes from the plasma components of the embryo. Later, as the organs of the embryo mature, there are other sources, such as the fetus's urine, the respiratory system, the gastrointestinal tract, the umbilical cord, and the placenta. Where does the word *amniotic* come from? It is an ancient term from the Chinese Yin Yang theory of medicine. The ancient characters for *Yin* and *Yang* are similar—they are homophones representing the beginning of human life, which is inseparable from the sun. Therefore, the origin of human life is called amniotic fluid. Thus, the *yangshui* became a symbol of the beginning of life, the birthplace of birth. Actually, amniotic fluid should be called *Yang water* to represent summers in Zhengyang, which are long, hot, oppressive, wet, and overcast.

Emboli are small solids that block blood vessels, or droplets that bubble into the blood circulation and block blood vessels. An amniotic fluid embolism refers to one that occurs during the second or third trimesters of labor or during or after delivery. Amniotic fluid can contain fetal hair, keratinized epithelium, fetal fat, meconium, dander, and other tangible substances that pass through the uterine placenta or cervix into the maternal blood. If any of these materials block circulation, severe complications such as acute pulmonary embolism, anaphylactic shock, disseminated intravascular coagulation, renal failure, and sudden death can occur.

Recent studies suggest that AFE is mainly an anaphylactic reaction caused by amniotic fluid entering the maternal circulation, which makes maternal antigens on the fetus produce a series of allergic reactions. It is a rare, not fully understood obstetric emergency. Most obstetricians have never seen an AFE case during their entire careers. The disorder was first described in 1941 as the fifth most common cause of maternal mortality. However, the high mortality rate seen in AFE cases, at greater than 86%, places the disorder in a category of serious and dangerous obstetric complications, in which 25% to 50% of patients die within 1 hour, making it one of the main causes of maternal death. A number of patients successfully treated still have brain injury, often due to hypoxia, and are left with damaged nervous system sequelae.

Under normal circumstances, amniotic fluid is enclosed in the amniotic sac. Because of the placental barrier between the mother and fetus, amniotic fluid is not in contact with the maternal circulatory system. However, the placental barrier may be injured during childbirth, or it may have been injured at some other time, causing a gap to occur and allowing amniotic fluid to enter the maternal system. If placental barrier defects are present, amniotic fluid, especially if it contains meconium and mucus, may induce AFE. The symptoms, prognosis, and treatments have important relationships. Was the AFE treated in time? Membrane rupture can occur postpartum or, more commonly, during full-term childbirth; it can also be seen with midterm induction or forceps curettage. China's statistics indicate that AFE mostly occurs up to two hours before delivery and within 30 minutes after delivery. It also occurs with amniocentesis, abortion, induced abortion, and closed abdominal injury. Seventy percent of AFE cases occur during the delivery process, 11% occur with vaginal delivery, and 19% occur after C-section. Embolism usually requires the following conditions: increased pressure in the amniotic cavity (from uterine contractions, including ankylosing uterine contraction); membrane rupture (67% of patients have prematurely ruptured membranes, while 33% have self-ruptured membranes); and cervical or uterine injury at open veins or sinusoids. AFE occurrences usually have the following characteristics: premature membrane rupture, including artificial membrane rupture; contractions that are too strong; improper oxytocin administration; and early placenta previa.

A statistical analysis performed in the US found that the incidence of AFE increases with age, certain ethnic origins, parity, previous abortion, previous obstetric disease, weight gain, hypertension, pregnancy with twins, delivery-route problems, and prolonged labor. Studies have not shown a relationship between AFE and oxytocin use, but AFE may be related to uterine contractions. When AFE is caused by pulmonary vascular disease, amniotic fluid components are not entirely the cause; however, amniotic fluid entrance into the blood after the release of some vasoactive substances is an important factor. In AFE cases, 78% of fetal membranes rupture, 33% of which rupture naturally and 67% of which rupture artificially. Use of an intrauterine pressure catheter has been found to have a certain relationship, with AFE occurring within 3 minutes after employment of this device. Additionally, 41% of AFE patients have a history of drug allergy or specific response, the majority of cases occurring when fetuses are male (67%).

Morbidity statistics have been less clear. Information collected using the medical library at the University of Florida were wide ranging, with some data indicating that 1 AFE death occurred in 8,000 to 80,000 births, and other data indicating that 4 to 6 AFE deaths occurred in 100,000 births. Because the diagnostic criteria are not very clear, the statistics vary widely, probably in the range of 1 death in 3,000 to 1 death in 30,000 births. The figures given in a 2007 study are from 20,464 births. US epidemiological statistics and international statistics estimate the incidence of AFE to be 1 case per 8,000 to 30,000 births. The true incidence is unknown because of inaccurate diagnoses and inconsistent reporting of nonfatal cases. In 2011, AFE was the leading cause of death during childbirth in Germany [14]. In Australia, AFE was cited as the leading direct cause of maternal death. Estimates range from 1 in 8,000 to 1 in 80,000 births [15]. In the United Kingdom, incidence is estimated at 1.9 to 7.7 in 100,000 births [16]. It is generally considered to occur in 1 in 6,000 to 1 in 12,000 cases. I agreed with Dr. Lu, the director of obstetrics and gynecology in Shenzhen City Central Hospital, that about 1 to 2 AFE cases per year occurred there. That hospital delivered around 500 newborns each month thirty-two years ago. Data show that the mortality rate is from 60% to 90%, with a mortality rate of 86% in the US. However, according to my experience, AFE mortality rate is closer to 90%, or even 100%. Much depends on when

AFE occurs during pregnancy, the amount of amniotic fluid that enters the mother's system, and the amniotic fluid turbidity, which is somewhat similar to the way that the extent of a building's damage from seawater influx during a hurricane is dependent on the intensity of the hurricane. Of course, our conclusion was based only on an estimate.

The high mortality rate for AFE, at 100%, is not absolute. As with airplane crashes, someone occasionally survives. *Obstetrics and Gynecology* (8th Ed.) indicates that the AFE death rate is 60% but generally could be as high as 80%! Of course, the mortality rate is very much linked to the level of medical care by the hospital staff and medical equipment available. Complications from childbirth that were previously more common in rural areas are beginning to occur in top hospitals in both China and the US. These hospitals with the world's best doctors and state-of-the-art medical equipment are often at a loss. I spoke about AFE with an Ob-Gyn whose name for the disorder was *Death*. Currently the medical profession finds it difficult to offer a detailed explanation of AFE pathogenesis. In general, it is thought that the following problems primarily contribute to this disorder: (1) amniotic pressure is too high; (2) sinusoids are open; (3) increased premature or artificial rupture of membranes occurs; (4) contractions are too strong, or oxytocin has been improperly administered; (5) early placental dissection, placenta previa, uterine rupture, or surgical production of AFE occurs; (6) stillbirth occurs (stillbirth increases AFE incidence because amniotic fluid enters the maternal circulation when fetal membranes are broken, a strong uterine contraction occurs, blood vessels open and allow a path to the endocervical and uterine veins, marginal veins of the placenta sinus open, damaged uterine sinusoids rupture further, and cervix becomes lacerated); (7) multiple organs are injured, and acute respiratory system failure occurs (DIC and other pathological changes often cause the mother to go into shock and have acute renal tubular necrosis, extensive hemorrhagic hepatic necrosis, and hemorrhage of the lungs and spleen).

Hemorrhage and acute liver and renal failure are the most common clinical manifestations; they are known as mutiple-system organ failure (MSOF), with almost 100% mortality when more than two vital organs fail to function simultaneously or sequentially. The pathophysiology of this is that the amniotic fluid moves into the maternal blood circulation, the tangible substances in the pulmonary arterioles and capillaries form an embolism, and the vagus nerve is excited, causing reflex pulmonary vasoconstriction, thus pulmonary hypertension, resulting in reduced lung perfusion and ventilation, blood flow imbalance, lung hypoxia, increased alveolar capillary permeability, fluid exudation, pulmonary edema, and pulmonary hemorrhage, leading to respiratory failure. Due to right ventricular drainage obstruction, acute right heart failure occurs, causing reduced left ventricular blood volume and leading to circulatory failure. Meconium, fetal fat, and other tangible substances in amniotic fluid are allergens, and upon entering the maternal circulatory system, they immediately cause anaphylactic shock and pulmonary hypertension.

In cases in which AFE caused sudden death, forensic experts found that the pathological changes were mainly seen in the pulmonary blood vessels. Although no specific changes were observed with the naked eye, microscopically, in both the pulmonary blood vessels and capillary cavity, keratinized epithelial cells were the main feature. Sometimes meconium and vellus hair were visible. The most common causes of sudden death were secondary vaginal bleeding and acute hemorrhagic shock caused by DIC, followed by AFE of the pulmonary arteries, which caused reflex vasospasm, pulmonary hypertension, heart failure, and respiratory failure. Death of some patients may have been due to visible components of amniotic fluid that caused allergic reactions and anaphylactic shock.

Short delivery time can also result in postpartum death, including after C-section. In rapid-onset cases, a high fatality rate has been observed, with sudden death occurring in about 67% of patients in 30 minutes to one hour. If a mother has sudden cardiac and pulmonary dysfunction during the delivery process, along with shock, and it is difficult to stop the vaginal bleeding, one should first consider AFE as the cause. At autopsy, pulmonary amniotic fluid components, especially keratinized epithelial cell material, is the necessary forensic identifier for AFE. Because AFE occurs during the delivery process, which is especially common with fetal disorders, the disorder can be diagnosed even if the body of the deceased was later contaminated. A primary pulmonary embolism caused by an amniotic epithelial cell mass is the main cause of respiratory failure and patient death.

CHAPTER 11
Deafening Silence
静处惊雷

NOTICE THE DEAFENING SILENCE of AFE. Amid its noiselessness comes the crash of thunder. It is characterized by a quiet, rapid development with no warning. It advances as softly as a rabbit, but then with an overwhelming pressure, a thunderous attack begins like a whistling storm. AFE behaves like a soldier, trained in *The Art of War* techniques, who uses the surprise attack on the unprepared. This disorder, which occurs suddenly, rapidly, like lightning, is extremely dangerous and has been referred to as obstetric death. It is estimated that maternal death from AFE can occur in minutes to hours. Approximately one-third of patients die within half an hour after onset, and another one-third die within an hour.

Chronic embolism, with only some bleeding and without rapid breathing or shortness of breath, is not a typical clinical manifestation. Almost all the patients I dealt with 32 years ago had simultaneous shortness of breath and postpartum hemorrhage. As mentioned above, one of the major features of AFE is rapid onset. Therefore, the major point is to react quickly, as it is a death race; the embolism should be caught as soon as possible. The patient will begin to pull back, her blood pressure will suddenly drop, and then she will become unconscious. The first suspicion should be AFE. Amniotic fluid embolism moves systemically, causing a variety of clinical manifestations, and if one waits until the clinical manifestations support the diagnosis, then it is too late. One must realize the essence of the phenomenon and act. The available response time is very short, so the treatment time should be similar in length to the reaction time of the *Swordsman* Dugu Jiu Jian—because, as he knows, "The enemy takes the first opportunity after his arrival."

CHAPTER 12
A Wandering Phantom
幽灵游荡

HOW MANY PREGNANT WOMEN and infants have died because of the invisible killer AFE, and how many lives have been ruined since humans appeared on the earth seven million years ago? One cannot be elegant when discussing this topic. So far, there is no literature that gives complete statistics. Many women have lost their precious lives to propagate the species. Although medical advances have made it possible to save patients with many high-risk conditions, AFE is an exception. The probability that a pregnant woman will have AFE is 1 in 12,000, but when it occurs, the death rate is a chilling 60% to 80%, or even 100% in some backward areas.

Since 2000, many medical controversies involving AFE have been described. Some women, after difficult rescues, have been able to come back from the *Ghosts' Gate*, but sometimes doctors are not proficient enough to save their patients. In maternal-death cases, family members often choose to appeal to the courts and may receive compensation in varying amounts. Some refuse to accept the verdict, while others settle the case with the hospital. The following are some of the AFE cases that occurred in China.

In August 2014, a maternal death occurred in Xiangtan County Maternal and Child Health Hospital in Hunan Province. The Xiangtan County Health Department said that the patient had died of AFE after 9 hours of rescue efforts. After her death, relatives submitted claims against the hospital in the amount of 1.2 million Yuan. The hospital was willing to pay about 500,000 Yuan. The rescue process for that case is described below.

At 6:10 a.m. on August 10, the pregnant woman arrived at Xiangtan County Maternal and Child Health Hospital for childbirth. At 12:05 p.m., a male baby was delivered. The mother began to vomit and choke. The initial diagnosis of AFE was made. At 2:20 p.m., the hospital issued a written notice of critical illness to family members. The patient's husband, Ryu, signed the form. At around 5:00 p.m., her uterus was removed. The multidimensional rescue failed, and maternal death occurred at 9:30 p.m.

The local media reported that, at around 11 p.m., the husband, having remained at the hospital, attempted to learn of his wife's condition, but no one responded to him. He ultimately opened the operating room door himself and discovered that all the doctors and nurses had already left the room.

The hospital reported that, at 9:40 p.m., the business department's chief informed the patient's cousin Zhang of her death. At around 11:00 p.m., the relatives of the deceased were reportedly out of control, exhibiting aggressive behavior. To avoid conflict between themselves and the family, the medical staff waited in the room next to the operating room. The patient's body had been placed on an operating table, with no staff remaining in the operating room.

In July 2014, one New Oriental Company staff member died of AFE in a hospital in Yunnan Province. The family members took the hospital to court. That case is described below.

At 2:00 p.m., on July 13, 2014, the pregnant woman entered the maternity ward of the Yunnan Province hospital. At 5:00 p.m., a doctor asked one of her family members to sign a statement of critical illness. The patient was transferred to the Red Cross Hospital at 1:30 a.m. on July 14. At 2:20 p.m., the mother was dead, and the newborn was in crisis. The patient's husband believed there were problems with the hospital's diagnosis and rescue attempt; he asserted that the hospital did not consider AFE as a possible diagnosis. However, a hospital representative responded by saying that doctors had actively treated the patient for AFE at the beginning of the delivery process and during the rescue effort.

In March 2014, in Guangdong Foshan, a pregnant woman's death occurred after medical mediation failed to save her from AFE, and her family resorted to legal prosecution. The rescue process began at 10:40 a.m. on March 1. The doctor began intravenous infusion of oxytocin. At around noon, the patient had convulsions and cyanosis. At 12:27 p.m., the hospital required family members to sign a form to allow C-section. At 2 p.m., the patient was sent to ICU for further care. At 6:35 p.m., the patient was declared dead. The fetus was declared clinically dead at 1:10 p.m. Relatives suspected that maternal death was a result of oxytocin injection. Hospital administration questioned why the patient had not been transferred to experts for treatment or experts had not been consulted. The hospital claimed that AFE rather than oxytocin had led to the patient's death. Also, experts had indeed arrived at the hospital at around the time of her death. The Guangdong Medical Commission and

Gaoming District Health Department helped co-ordinate the rescue effort, but their mediation failed. Family members resorted to legal procedures to resolve liability and compensation issues.

· In February 2014, a woman named Dazhou Sichuan agreed to terminate her fetus, but she died of AFE nevertheless. Because the infant would have been abnormal, Dazhou Cannes Hospital proposed to abort it, and family members agreed. The patient was given mifepristone tablets to ultimately protect her own safety. At 6 p.m. on February 22, her situation was unstable. At 9 p.m., she vomited blood and began hemorrhaging. At 2:00 p.m. the next day, the hospital, having no rescue equipment, made a call to have the patient transferred to the Dazhou Integrative Medicine Hospital. After the transfer and rescue attempts, maternal death occurred.

Family members thought that giving mifepristone to the patient had been appropriate but that the dosage was excessive, and that the hospital delayed the rescue effort. They raised many questions and asked the hospital to compensate them with 800,000 Yuan. Emotions were out of control, and the family was responsible for a head wound to Mr. Lee, the vice president of Dazhou Cannes Hospital. The hospital claimed there had been no problem with the medication but that AFE had resulted from the patient's own health condition. The hospital said it was not responsible for damage caused by the drugs administered and that no medical accident had occurred. The hospital was not willing to give more than one Yuan of monetary compensation. Personnel from the local health bureau and law enforcement came forward to organize mediation between the hospital and family. Because both parties have disproportionately suffered, no agreement has yet been reached. Both parties are willing to seek judicial arbitration.

In July 2013, a woman named Zhu died from AFE in Zhejiang Shangyu. The hospital eventually paid 200,000 Yuan in compensation. Medical intervention began on the morning of July 14 after the patient arrived at the Shangyu Mother and Child Health Hospital. At about noon, she said she was unwell and requested a C-section. The hospital said her situation was normal and that she could have a natural birth. She was sent to the emergency room at about 1 p.m. At 5 p.m., her death occurred. The patient's husband said his wife had been deceased for about 8 hours, yet the hospital would not allow family members to view her body. Also, family members claimed that after the woman had died, the attending physicians left. The hospital said that at about 8 p.m. on July 14, staff informed the family that the patient's body had been moved to the funeral parlor. Additionally, the hospital spokesperson said, "The attending physician has been on the scene," and, "There was no disappearance by medical staff." After mediation, as an appeasement, the hospital paid the deceased patient's family a total of 200,000 Yuan. Family members accepted the mediation. Both doctors and family differed on the amount of compensation due. After the autopsy results, judicial proceedings for the case began.

In June 2009, in Wu Li County, Henan, AFE occurred in a patient, and the hospital was required to pay compensation of 50,000 Yuan to the patient's dependents. The rescue process began as early as 7:10 a.m. on June 1 in the delivery ward of the Maternal and Child Health Hospital. By 8:25 a.m., convulsions, respiratory arrest, and other symptoms occurred, and the hospital began rescue efforts. After 2 hours, both the mother and child had died from AFE. At the hospital, 50 to 60 workers were besieged for a few hours by the patient's family members, most of them being hit about the head. Healthcare employees were bleeding; some had pierced eardrums. The hospital president himself had been forced to kneel and grovel before the dead patient. The doctor had advised the family to agree to a C-section, but that had been rejected by them, and they instead insisted on physician-assisted labor combined with traditional delivery. After mediation, it was concluded that no medical accident occurred, but rather there had been negligence on the part of the patient's family. The Maternal and Child Health Hospital gave a one-time compensation of 50,000 Yuan to the family. Family members who had caused injuries to the healthcare staff were detained.

In September 1999, in Beijing, a death due to AFE was the reason the Xichang District Exhibition Road Hospital gave compensation of 158,000 Yuan to the patient's family. At 7:45 p.m. on September 9, the woman gave birth to a baby girl. At 1:30 a.m., because of hemorrhage, her womb was excised, with the consent of family members. At 4:30 a.m., maternal death occurred. The patient's husband thought the hospital should be held responsible for her death, and he appealed to hospital administration for compensation of 250,000 Yuan, based on his various losses. The doctor who attended the rescue effort concluded that the patient had died of

AFE. The hospital claimed that it "had never before seen this kind of case."

At the trial, on December 20, 2000, the Xicheng District Central Court announced its verdict: The hospital had a responsibility to treat patients with care, and when patients and their families experienced losses because of improper treatment, the hospital was at fault and should bear the main liability for compensation. The court ruled against the defendant and the Exhibition Road Hospital compensated the plaintiff with 158,000 Yuan.

In November 1998, in Changling County, Jilin Province, in the Central Hospital, a maternal death from AFE occurred. Family members sued the hospital, eventually receiving compensation of 280,000 Yuan. The rescue process began at 2:20 p.m. on November 6. Nine hours later, the mother gave birth to a baby boy, who was diagnosed with cerebral palsy. The mother died two hours later. The patient's husband believed that the hospital, during the process of natural childbirth, made an error that resulted in the death of his wife. He asked the hospital to provide compensation of 28,000 Yuan. The hospital claimed that the death was due to AFE and postpartum complications and therefore was a normal death. At trial, the Changling County and SongYuan City Medical Accreditation Committee identified the death as not being a medical accident; whereas, the Jilin Province Medical Accreditation Committee stated that "the incident was a two-level medical and technical accident."

In May 2014, a maternal AFE case occurred in Zhanjiang, Guangdong Province. The mother and child were saved during the rescue process, which included removal of the uterus and administration of a large number of intravenous infusions, equivalent to a whole-body exchange transfusion. Upon hearing from the Wuchuan Maternity and Child Health Care Hospital that his wife was in critical condition, the husband signed a letter of informed consent. When he first learned that his wife was a rare, high-risk patient, it was his hope that she would be treated by doctors at that particular hospital.

In December 2012, in Hainan Sanya, an older woman was saved from death. On the evening of December 15, the 43-year-old pregnant woman arrived at the Sanya City Central Hospital. Her pregnancy was complicated by high blood pressure, placental abruption, and another high-risk disorder, severe AFE. The hospital decisively performed a hysterectomy, resulting in a successful rescue.

In August 2004, in Jiangsu Yancheng, during the removal of an amniotic fluid embolus, a uterine blood transfusion was administered to the patient, at a cost of nearly 30,000 Yuan. To save her, a suction machine was employed, and oxytocin and 19 ampules of albumin were administered. The entire treatment cost nearly 80,000 Yuan. After the delivery of twin boys, it was noted that the oldest boy's head had an indention; also his eyes were dull in appearance. The mother was unconscious for seven days, but then her condition improved. The family thought the large medical bills were a result of their having been misled by doctors and therefore that the hospital should assume some responsibility. The hospital claimed the patient's condition occurred because of AFE, that it had done all it could to save the mother and infants, and that the husband, Mr. Song, should thank the doctor and hospital. The medical expenses at the hospital were completely standard.

On August 19, 2014, CCTV-News reported that 53 bags of blood were successfully delivered in Shanghai for the rescue of a woman with AFE.

On August 6, 2015, the Shandong Commercial Daily News reported that blood was urgently needed for a patient with AFE; subsequently, lines of thousands of people began forming for blood donations in Jinan. On August 10, the Sichuan city newspaper reported that the young woman Yang Jingni had died, but the public did not get the bad news and continued to donate blood.

At Xingguo County Central Hospital in June 2017, a placenta previa was successfully treated during C-section on a pregnant woman with AFE.

On September 12, 2017, the Hunan Shaodong Central Hospital successfully saved a patient with AFE. Transfusions totaling 4,600 cc of blood were given during the rescue.

Researchers at the Washington University Institute for Health Statistics and Evaluation wrote in the weekly medical journal *The Lancet* that, over the past decade, the US was one of only eight countries in which the maternal mortality rate had risen. The other seven countries included Afghanistan, Greece, and several African and Central American countries. In 2013, 18.5 maternal deaths per 100,000 births occurred in the US (compared with only half that number in other developed countries, including France), bringing the total number of deaths to nearly 800, which was higher than that in Saudi Arabia and Canada.

The US maternal mortality rate has more than doubled and is now greater than twice that in the United Kingdom. The US ranks at sixtieth place out of 180 countries, up sharply from its twenty-second place in 1990, and comparable to China's position at fifty-seventh place. The reasons for the increase in the US are not yet fully understood; however, doctors state that several factors are involved. First, maternal mortality rates have been improving year by year. Second, an increase in pregnant women who have diseases that cause high-risk pregnancies, such as hypertension and diabetes, has occurred. Additionally, obesity and its associated diseases are important causes of maternal mortality in the US. High-risk conditions can be associated with the increased mortality from AFE. China and the US report huge differences in recognition of maternal mortality and resultant compensation. With so many maternal deaths in the US each year, why are family members' reactions not producing an effect toward curing it? The answer is because of comprehensive laws, independent investigations, and the insurance system. By observing the many ongoing domestic medical disputes, one can conclude that responsibility is rarely recognized and compensation results are not usually satisfactory.

According to a *Los Angeles Times* report in March 2014, a Chinese woman in California died from hemorrhage after giving birth to a child. Later, an Orange County court ruled that the woman's husband, Yuanda Hong, and her two children would be awarded 5.2 million US dollars, equaling more than 30 million Yuan. The reason given was that the Chinese physician who attended to her was accused of serious negligence. In China, however, hospitals and doctors seldom take full responsibility; although, in cases of maternal medical disputes, doctors and hospitals have been shown to have a clear causal relationship with mortality. As to the amount of compensation, the two countries are even farther apart.

In 2013, a fetal-death case occurred in Jiangxi Province. The court directed the hospital to assume part of the responsibility; the compensation requested was 30,000 Yuan. The husband had refused to sign a form that listed death as a possible outcome of his wife's surgery. In the initial verdict, the court stated that the Beijing Capital Medical University subsidiary Beijing Chaoyang Hospital bore no responsibility, but after taking into account the actual facts of the case, the Chaoyang Hospital was directed to pay the plaintiff 100,000 Yuan in compensation, which was a high amount.

The amount of compensation due to a patient or patient's family is to a large extent based on the the hospital's liability, which depends on the negligence. The basic elements of constitutional law are similar throughout the world, a primary element being whether the doctor or medical institution is at fault and a secondary element being the causal relationship between negligence and personal injury. In mainstream countries, standards of judgment for medical negligence are similar. In China, instructors of the various medical disciplines frequently reference US and European Union (EU) standards. Their judgment standards are primarily in line with the rest of the world. However, in regard to causal relationships, China's position is different from that of other countries, especially developed countries. Most countries first consider the legal implications of causation by determining whether the injury would have occurred without the negligence. If that were the case, what would have been the probability of avoiding the injury?

In the 2013 Beijing incident, for example, the court presumed that the fetus would have died before delivery because of AFE even if the attending physician had monitored the patient from the beginning and had continued the observation to the end of the case. A criterion that was used was that the death was 100% causal, with the hospital at fault, because the attending doctor could have prevented the death, as there was a greater-than-50% probability of death occurring without his care. Also, because of China's regulations on medical malpractice, courts consider primary maternal diseases to be important. Postpartum hemorrhages almost always are caused by primary diseases such as placental abruption, coagulopathy, and AFE. If the judgement criteria are followed, doctors and hospitals must take full responsibility for injuries that are less likely to occur. Another important difference in China is the lack of independent investigation. Settlement of medical disputes is difficult because the industry is small and the doctors know each another. Judgment would be less difficult if it were not affected by such human relationships. Also, medical records are often incomplete and may not be kept in storage; thus, thorough, effective investigations may be difficult to carry out and may have to be settled partly through guesswork.

The general public in China is dissatisfied with most medical institutions because of the executive administration. Government influence is the reason that hospitals usually win cases brought against them by patients. In the US, hospitals are not subject to as much government interference, and they guarantee patients more personal rights. Policies, terms, and conditions are meant to benefit individuals. Patients are considered to be much more vulnerable than hospitals and doctors, and because they generally lack the medical knowledge possessed by doctors, they may be given discretionary compensation considered to be "humane and reasonable." In the US, the median amount of medical malpractice compensation given to the plaintiff is $230,000, and out-of-court settlements have exceeded $120,000. However, when news media become involved, compensation may be seen that is in the millions or even in the tens of millions of dollars. A few years ago, a US boy who suffered serious head injuries because of a hospital's negligence received $97 million in compensation.

Such huge compensation amounts do not greatly damage doctors and hospitals. In the US, doctors, including anesthesiologists, and even nurses buy their own liability insurance. When malpractice occurs, the insurance company will deal with it and compensate for it as necessary. Annual medical-liability insurance premiums of most American doctors account for about 10% of their annual incomes, with premiums for Ob-Gyns accounting for 15% to 18% of their annual incomes. Thus, doctors and hospitals do not attempt to reduce their liability for compensation.

In 2010, Melanie Pritchard survived AFE in Phoenix, Arizona. She wrote of this experience in the book *The Day I Died*. It was reported that she died to overcome her pain. Her expected date of childbirth was July 28, 2010, and at midnight on that date, she suddenly felt abdominal pain and dizziness; her husband then drove her to the hospital. Upon arriving there, her blood pressure and heartbeat were found to be abnormal. Also, the heart rate of her unborn child dropped sharply, and not long afterward, Melanie's heart stopped beating. She was taken to the operating room where the doctor tried to save both her and her infant by performing a C-section. During surgery, Melanie was clinically dead for 10 minutes because of massive AFE. During CPR, with defibrillation applied 4 times, a healthy baby girl was born. What seemed even more miraculous was that Melanie herself was "resurrected."

In September 2012, a pregnant British woman named Michelle suffered from AFE. With the help of an AFE foundation in the United Kingdom, she survived the disorder. In Zhangqiu City, China, in October 2013, Shandong Maternal and Child Health Hospital successfully saved a pregnant woman who had AFE. Also in 2013, the Second Affiliated Hospital of Nanchang University successfully treated a woman with a dangerous case of AFE.

CHAPTER 13
Take Precautions
未雨绸缪

ACCORDING TO A WELL-KNOWN saying, "Being prepared ensures success, and being unprepared brings about failure." With improvements in perinatal care, AFE prevention and treatment have been raised to a higher level. Precautionary measures are the key to preventing medical complications. During prenatal examinations, I strongly recommend making risk assessments to help keep all parties vigilant. Small things can become large, as is explained by the familiar proverb "When soil accumulates, it becomes a hill; when water accumulates, it becomes a river." I also recommend that pregnant women do the following:

(1) Enhance their physical strength by practicing guided Qigong. To perform Tai Chi, I recommend 24 simplified movements of Taijiquan, Baduanjin (8 sections of movement), Huatuo's Five Animal Exercise (without straining too much), and Yi Jin Jing.

(2) Practice yoga, meditation, and relaxation, and listen to music, especially classical music. Music and healing have been inextricably linked since ancient times. In Greek mythology, Apollo was in charge of both medicine and music. In the early twentieth century, music therapy was gradually accepted by society. A patient's psychology and physiology will improve with music during medical procedures. Playing music in the delivery room can produce positive results. It is

recommended that women, during pregnancy and after delivery, listen to classical music, or any beautiful, melodious music, for half an hour each day. This will be conducive to good health for not only the fetus and infant but also for the mother. A relaxed mood makes relaxed nerves.

(3) Learn how to "detoxify" the soul and "avoid being led around by the nose." Before bed each night a pregnant woman should recall three things she is grateful for, which will increase her happiness and which in turn will increase her sensitivity toward good things and help her maintain a positive mood. Chinese medicine teaches that "If one is upright inside, evil cannot intimidate. Malevolence flows away, becoming only empty air." This viewpolnt opens up the paths necessary for preventing and treating AFE.

(4) Strive to absorb more sunshine at the same time every day during pregnancy. The sun is the best vitamin-D activator. Also, sunshine speeds up blood circulation and promotes calcium absorption, preventing postpartum osteoporosis. There are many surprises in store for mother and baby. Having healthy tendons in the arms and legs is worth promoting.

(5) Pay attention to the details of life and do more exercises, such as hip lifts, which can improve blood circulation and keep hemorrhoids from forming. During pregnancy, because of endocrine changes, including in progesterone, muscle relaxin will increase, making smooth muscle relaxation easier, and intestinal peristalsis will decrease, causing constipation to occur more easily. Also, because of the decrease in intestinal peristalsis, the amount of water absorbed will increase, causing constipation. Up to 80% of

pregnant women will have constipation problems far worse than in the average person, and of these constipated pregnant women, about 76% will have perhaps two or three hemorrhoids.

(6) Pay attention to drinking-water safety. If lead levels in the human body are too high, the nervous, digestive, hematopoietic, and renal systems will be seriously endangered. The effect on a baby's intelligence and physical development can be especially serious.

(7) Take measures to achieve harmony with nature, peace and unity in yin and yang, balance in the five elements, and an enhanced physical condition; these will help prevent AFE.

(8) During childbirth, strive to adhere to this advice: "Sleep between the contractions, tolerate the pain, and be slow to give birth."

The theory of the Yellow Emperor, Huangdi Neijing, was that "We originate from tranquil nothingness, and if we keep within the spirit, sickness never enters." The following high-risk patients should be particularly vigilant: (1) Mothers who are more than 35 years of age; they have higher rates of AFE; the older the mother, the higher the rate. (2) Mothers who have higher birth numbers; e.g., mothers expecting second, third, or fourth babies (and so on) have higher rates of AFE; the higher the birth number, the higher the rate. (3) Patients who have early placental dissection; during reproduction, if early placental exfoliation occurs, amniotic fluid may contain fetal cells, fetal fat, or meconium, and the flow of this material through the placental veins into the maternal bloodstream will increase the possibility of AFE. (4) Patients whose fetuses have died in their wombs; the longer fetuses have been dead, the higher the risk for AFE. (5) Patients who have fetal-distress phenomenon; because of fetal distress, amniotic fluid will often contain meconium, causing intense pain and a greater risk for AFE; the incidence of AFE will be relatively high. (6) Patients who were given oxytocin; intense pain may result; patients are also more likely to have AFE. (7) Patients who are pregnant with boy babies; some think these women have an increased possibility of having AFE, but no true data exists. (8) Women who are diagnosed with depression; research shows that in today's society women are more likely to suffer from severe depression, and those who have depression have a higher risk of dying at any time. Perinatal depression can occur before or after childbirth. Previously, most attention was given to postpartum depression; now prenatal depression has also become a concern, as has the patient's psychological state during delivery. Pregnant women should not neglect their psychological health. Timely introspection and prevention are key.

Are there ways to decrease the risk factors of AFE? If prenatal precautionary measures are taken, patients can be saved. Doctors should make patients aware of the following information that can help prevent AFE: (1) B-mode ultrasound inspection can diagnose 90% of placenta previa cases, and childbirth monitoring devices are useful for the early detection of placental abruption. These two abnormalities may be the cause of AFE. (2) To protect prenatal health, early detection of pregnancy-induced hypertension is essential. Once high blood pressure occurs, edema and proteinuria can follow. Treatment must be actively carried out to avoid these symptoms. Women of age 30 and older may have premature membrane rupture in the uterus or cervical dysplasia, predisposing them to AFE. These induced factors should be closely observed, and the patient should be made aware of possible AFE and educated about C-section, placenta previa, early stripping of placenta, and so on. (3) Patients should promptly inform the doctor of abnormal symptoms noticed during the delivery process. These include chest tightness, irritability, chills, and other uncomfortable feelings. This is important because it gives doctors more time to take necessary actions. (4) Timely C-section should be performed if AFE symptoms occur during the first labor stage because the fetus cannot be delivered immediately otherwise. Although the condition may improve with medical action, the cause will not have been removed, and the possibility of deterioration is present. C-section will bring about delivery quickly and reduce the risk of uterine rupture. (5) Birth trauma, uterine rupture, cervical laceration, and other conditions should be avoided by following all precautions. (6) A credible hospital should be selected for prenatal care and delivery.

Obstetricians should take note of the following points: (1) Childbirth should not be delayed too long, allowing contractions to become too strong. Very strong pressure from intrauterine contraction can cause rupture of the lower uterus and allow amniotic fluid to pass through the gap into the maternal bloodstream. Appropriate sedatives should be administered to inhibit uterine contractility and reduce contractions. (2) Oxytocin indications should be strictly observed and controlled; oxytocin should be used rationally. During the labor process, if uterine contractions are too strong, sedative drugs should be administered in a timely manner to weaken contractions and prevent uterine rupture. (3) C-section indications should be strictly observed and controlled. In particular, cephalopelvic disproportion, if present, should be detected as soon as possible to avoid uterine rupture. Early detection of pathological uterine rupture can help avert the crisis of AFE. (4) To strictly control artificial membrane rupture, ruffled gauze pads should be used to protect the incision edge, and the amniotic membrane should be pierced to protect the open vessels at the uterine incision. Artificial membrane rupture should not be concurrent with stripping, so that any damage to the small vessels of the cervix will be minimal and contractions will not cause them to rupture. (5) During a midterm induced abortion, when the first membrane rupture occurs and amniotic fluid begins to flow, a clamp should be used to stop the fluid, and oxytocin should be administered. (6) In the second stage, to avoid abdominal pain, adequate pressure should be applied to the patient, without using excessive force. (7) Close observation should occur during the fourth labor stage, which may or may not include shortness of breath, dyspnea, chills, and other symptoms. A timely detection of bleeding should occur, and notice should be taken whenever a symptom does not match the situation.

CHAPTER 14
Timely Diagnosis
及时诊断

A DOCTOR WORKING ON an AFE case should always be vigilant, remaining keenly aware and calm. Early diagnosis should occur, and quick, precise action should be taken to save the patient. The situation will be subject to chaos; thus, the staff must act decisively so as not to delay treatment. The patient must also have some medical knowledge. Amniotic fluid embolism should be suspected if, after induction of labor, membrane rupture or sudden unexplained dyspnea, cyanosis, or shock occurs. If DIC occurs, AFE is highly likely. However, the etiology is not easy to determine with preliminary diagnosis, which is only based on clinical manifestations. The treatment and rescue effort should be of immediate concern; further examination will confirm the diagnosis.

The common manifestations of AFE are as follows:

(1) A shock period, which occurs suddenly, presents sometimes with screaming, chills, twitching, purple coloration within a few seconds, breathing difficulties, chest tightness, irritability, and vomiting. Only a short period of time occurs before the shock state is entered. Most patients die quickly and with a small number of symptoms, including right heart failure, acute right ventricle enlargement, rapid heart rate, jugular vein engorgement, hepatomegaly, and tenderness. Some patients also have pulmonary edema,

coughing, slightly pink, foamy sputum, and lungs full of rales. Respiratory failure and coma follow.

(2) A bleeding period presents with a large amount of continuous postpartum vaginal hemorrhaging. The blood has not coagulated, and while the contractions occur, the bleeding continues. The body has a tendency toward extensive bleeding of the skin, mucous membranes, respiratory tract, digestive tract, urinary tract, incision wounds, and the puncture site. Ecchymoses and petechiae are evident.

(3) Renal failure occurs with oliguria, anuria, and uremia symptoms. Because of the long period of shock, renal microvascular embolism results from the renal tissue damage due to ischemia. Sometimes the three stages of incomplete delivery result in pulmonary hypertension. The effects seen postpartum are mainly due to coagulation disorders and are listed as follows: (A) pulmonary hypertension and pulmonary edema; acute right heart failure and peripheral circulatory failure; (B) anaphylactic shock; hypoxemia; (D) disseminated intravascular coagulation.

Amniotic fluid containing visible components causes blood to coagulate, a fibrin plug to form in the pulmonary circulation, and the pulmonary vascular channel to narrow, while the vagus nerve excitement causes pulmonary vasospasm and bronchial secretion. Pressure on pulmonary arterioles and microvasculature suddenly increases, leading to acute right heart failure. The amount of blood returning to the left atrium becomes significantly reduced, resulting in decreased left ventricular ejection, which is also caused by the circulatory failure resulting from low blood pressure. In addition, because the amniotic fluid meconium or other particulate matter may be recognized as allergens, AFE can result from anaphylaxis, which causes a condition similar to chills and a rapidly declining blood pressure or no blood pressure at all. Due to pulmonary hypertension, perfusion decreases so that a ventilation-blood flow imbalance occurs, along with acute respiratory failure and pulmonary edema, leading to severe systemic hypoxemia. The body tissues and vital organs are then in a dysfunctional state. Critical organ dysfunction, especially of lung, brain, and kidney, can lead to rapid maternal death. The diagnosis will be AFE with 50% concurrent DIC.

An increase in clotting factor occurs during pregnancy. Decreased fibrinolytic activity itself is a hypercoagulable state. Amniotic fluid is rich in thromboplastin; thus, once it enters the blood-stream, it can cause acute DIC. DIC is a temporary hypercoagulable state. During the original decline, which causes the fibrinolytic system to become activated, the blood is rapidly transferred from a hypercoagulable state to a fibrinolytic state, resulting in blood coagulation and severe postpartum hemorrhage. Amniotic fluid embolism is highly dangerous and requires urgent treatment, as maternal death can occur within minutes; therefore, if a pregnant woman suddenly begins to scream, has respiratory difficulties, bruising lips, blood pressure change, bleeding, shock, coma, and other symptoms, the doctor must be extremely vigilant for the possibility of AFE and must immediately begin the rescue effort. The doctor cannot wait for the test results or a clear diagnosis. Treatment must begin immediately. Early bloody sputum may appear, and the doctor may begin to hear wet rales and notice signs of pulmonary edema.

A radiograph will show a fan-shaped shadow in the hilar sector, and right heart enlargement. An electrocardiogram stimulating the right ventricle will indicate right atrial enlargement. Often, on viewing myocardial strain images and radioactive iodine (I-131) lung scans, perfusion defects may be seen, which are helpful in diagnosing the sudden decline in oxygen saturation that can often prompt pulmonary embolism. A CT and an MRI that show cerebrovascular changes have a higher diagnostic value. The exact diagnosis will be obvious from the vena cava blood sample. Amniotic fluid will be found in the squamous epithelium, and mucus, vellus hair, and other tangible substances in the arterioles and capillaries will be confirmed by autopsy. In recent years, squamous epithelial cells have been noted in blood films.

At routine examination and from laboratory test results of patients, the following have been noted: (1) Right ventricular EKGs show evidence of right atrial expansion; also, myocardial strain may be shown to be concurrent with tachycardia. (2) Chest radiographs may not show abnormalities, but 70% of patients have mild symptoms of pulmonary edema, with a diffuse bilateral shadow distributed around the hilar sector, and slightly enlarged lungs. (3) A sudden drop in oxygen saturation can often prompt pulmonary embolism. (4) Coagulation test results vary widely, with results dependent on the patient's survival time and the extent of clinical bleeding [Platelet count: $<100 \times 10^9$/L; Prothrombin time: >10 sec (which is diagnostic); Plasma fibrinogen: <1.5g/L;

Clotting observation (tests are performed in vitro, using a control of normal maternal blood; samples are observed for clot formation for 8 to 12 min; if low fibrinogen, blood coagulation will be diminished; blood may clot after 30 min; dispersion will show that platelets have been quite low, with secondary fibrinolysis): bleeding and clotting times will be extended; fibrin degradation products will be increased; and plasma protamine coagulation test (3P test) and ethanol gel tests will be positive.

Amniotic fluid embolism specificity can be evaluated in the following ways: (1) Amniotic fluid components may be detected in the circulatory system or in lung tissue. Because fetal tissue such as squamous cells, hair, and mucus can enter the bloodstream and cause pulmonary embolism and spasms, they are the diagnostic criteria for evaluating peripheral blood, uterine blood vessels, and lung tissue. (2) D-Sialyl-Tn (STn) antigen may be detected in serum and lung tissue using new immunological technology. Kobayashi and others have found that mucinous glycoprotein monoclonal antibody TKH-2 can recognize the amniotic fluid mucus glycoprotein oligosaccharide structure with immunoblotting techniques. TKH-2 detects very low concentrations of sTn antigen in meconium supernates. Antigens that can be recognized by TKH-2 are present not only in large quantities in meconium but also in clear amniotic fluid. Immunohistochemical detection of antigens by TKH-2 reaction is common in small intestine, colon, and respiratory tract epithelial cells. Radioimmunoassay of meconium-stained amniotic fluid and clear amniotic fluid can provide measurements of sTn antigen, with values for the former significantly higher than for the latter. STn antigen was found to be a characteristic component of meconium and amniotic fluid, accounting for about one-tenth of meconium. The origin of sTn antigen in amniotic fluid is still not very clear. Because of the expression of sTn antigen in the mucosal epithelium of the digestive and respiratory tracts, it is considered that, in addition to meconium being the main source of sTn antigen in amniotic fluid, some may come from respiratory tract mucus protein. The concentration of sTn antigen in the serum of women after pregnancy can vary. If meningitis occurs, the concentration of sTn antigen in serum (20.3 ± 15.4 U/mL) is slightly higher than in clear amniotic fluid (11.8 ± 5.6 U/mL). However, in serum of patients with AFE or AFE-like symptoms, the sTn antigen increases significantly (105.6 ± 59.0 U/mL). The radioimmuno-competition assay for quantitative determination of sTn antigen in serum has been shown to be a simple, sensitive, non-invasive method of diagnosing AFE, and it can be used in early diagnosis. Histological diagnosis after maternal death is still very important. Strong, positive immunohistochemical staining of lung tissue with TKH-2, which reveals significant positive staining of pulmonary vessels in patients with AFE or AFE-like symptoms, can be completely inhibited by submandibular gland mucus protein, indicating that it is immunospecific. (3) Tissue Anticoagulant Factor can be measured in the above-mentioned tangible components in amniotic fluid. It may not be the main cause of AFE; some humoral factors, such as tissue factor-like procoagulant substances, leukotrienes, and other similar substances, have very important roles.

About 40% of AFE occurs in patients who have fatal coagulopathy. The coagulation activity of Tissue Factor can be antagonized by Tissue Factor Protein, so it is theoretically possible to test for Tissue Factor in maternal blood as a basis for distinguishing other obstetric DICs. (4) The presence of mast cells in lung tissue is diagnostic for AFE. In recent years, researchers have described a mechanism in which the fetal components cause allergic reaction, leading to mast cell degranulation and subsequent histamine release. Trypsin and other agents can cause serious disease and physiological changes. Tryptase is a neutral protease that is a major component of T-cells and mast cell–secreting particles. Fineschi and others found, by special immunohistochemical detection of mast-cell tryptase in pulmonary circulatory tissue samples, that due to AFE and anaphylactic shock, the mast cell count in lung tissue was significantly increased. There was no difference between these patients and those who died of trauma. There was a significantly lower number of mast cells in the lung tissue of shock patients, compared to AFE and anaphylactic shock patients, who tested positive for pulmonary mast-cell tryptase with immunohistochemical testing.

Forensic identification points are important in AFE cases. AFE commonly occurs a short time after delivery. It can also occur during C-section or postpartum. Often rapid onset occurs, and there is a high fatality rate, with about two-thirds of patients dying suddenly after about 30 minutes to one hour. If, during the childbirth process, sudden cardiac and pulmonary dysfunction occur and shock and vaginal bleeding become difficult to reverse, one should immediately consider AFE as the probable cause. An autopsy that diagnoses AFE will show pulmonary amniotic fluid components, especially keratinized epithelial material. Even if a deceased patient's body has been contaminated, an autopsy will be able to show that entire organs were damaged; the heart and kidneys will be most damaged. Because of kidney hypoxia, urine will be decreased, and hematuria and azotemia will result from renal failure and death. Patients with brain hypoxia may have exhibited irritability, had convulsions, and become comatose. The exact diagnosis can be made from a sample of vena cava blood, which will include amniotic fluid with squamous epithelium, hair, and other tangible substances. Autopsy will confirm the presence of AFE in pulmonary arterioles or capillaries. As mentioned previously, squamous epithelial cells reportedly have been found in blood films.

CHAPTER 15
Differential Diagnosis
鉴别诊断

AFE CAN BE EASILY misdiagnosed as other disorders, such as uterine rupture:

(1) Uterine rupture. It may be caused by the following circumstances: (A) Natural conditions, such as the fetus blocking the pelvis stenosis; cephalopelvic disproportion; abnormal fetal position (such as incarcerated transverse position); fetal malformations (such as hydrocephalus); obstruction of the birth canal; other obstructions to labor that may overcome strong uterine contractions; lower uterine thinning; fetal exposure exceeding the maximum limit, which can occur at the weak, lower end of the umbilical support. (B) Improper use of uterine contraction devices; large doses of oxytocin, resulting in too-intense uterine contractions; first fetal exposure causing uterine rupture. (C) Rupture of surgical scar tissue on uterus (uterus contracting or stretching so significantly that the increased pressure causes rupture of a scar from previous surgery); previous C-section scar rupturing during late pregnancy (lower segment of a C-section rupturing incompletely, postpartum); pathological changes of uterine muscle wall (due to multiple births, curettage, history of uterine perforation, uterine teratogenesis, uterine hypoplasia, etc.) that increase the chance of uterine rupture. (D) Instrument trauma by midwife during vaginal delivery, especially with uterine inversion,

improper mechanical clamp use, or rough delivery.

(2) Early placental dissection. (A) Light type usually occurs with vaginal bleeding, often heavy bleeding; blood is dark red, and bleeding may be associated with mild abdominal pain or no obvious abdominal pain; on abdominal examination, uterus is soft, with no obvious tenderness or only mild, localized tenderness. (B) Heavy type occurs during hidden, excessive bleeding.

(3) Preeclampsia. Symptoms of convulsions, hypertension, edema, and proteinuria usually occur in prenatal, maternity, and postnatal periods, with no rupturing of membranes and no exhaling difficulties detected in lungs by auscultation; DIC lab test results are usually normal.

(4) Congestive heart failure. When there is a history of heart disease, there is an increased burden on the heart; patient suddenly has palpitations, shortness of breath, coughing, foamy sputum, and generally no convulsions, bleeding, or renal failure. After heart-medicine treatment, symptoms can be improved.

(5) Cerebrovascular incidence. Occurs in patients with a history of hypertension, headache, dizziness, sudden coma, and hemiplegia.

(6) Epilepsy. Patients often have a history of seizure; sometimes mental issues develop; patients generally have no bleeding, DIC, or renal failure.

(7) Other causes of non-DIC postpartum hemorrhage. A clear cause can generally be found; according to causes, hemorrhage can be divided into four categories: postpartum bleeding causing weak uterine contractions, placental retention,

lacerations of soft tissue in birth canal, and coagulation disorders.

(8) Thromboembolic disease. Patients often are in a hypercoagulable state; deep vein thrombosis (DVT) generally occurs without bleeding.

(9) Pregnancy complicated by acute suppurative cholangitis. Acute suppurative cholangitis is a disease of rapid development, serious complications, and high mortality rates; if not treated in a timely manner, patient will be prone to septic shock; early treatment is crucial; it has three typical characteristics: (A) It causes chills, fever, and confusion. (B) It is due to bile duct obstruction that causes inflammation and mostly persistent abdominal pain. (C) It is due to poor bile drainage and causes jaundice.

(10) Appendicitis during pregnancy. Occurs as complication from concurrent pericarditis perforation; often presents as severe lower-right abdominal pain with vomiting and diarrhea; no vaginal bleeding is present unless spontaneous abortion occurs; patient should be checked for obvious tenderness; whole-abdomen tenderness and rebound tenderness may occur as result of peripheral appendicitis; often tenderness point other than Mark's tenderness point is present; according to the month of pregnancy, tenderness point may be increased; as soon as possible, perform B-mode ultrasound inspection to diagnose appendicitis; perform surgery as soon as possible; otherwise, spontaneous abortion may occur, along with damage to patient's life.

(11) Pregnancy with asthma. Patients with history of asthma have breathing difficulties that are particularly evident with auscultation: asthma sounds in lungs, wet rales; no abnormal vaginal bleeding occurs; treatment with ammonia theophylline can have significant positive effect.

(12) Perinatal depression. Occurs before and after childbirth. Although attention has mostly been on postpartum depression, prenatal depression has also become a concern. Based on my long-term experience, I conclude that the psychological state of women in China during the prenatal (pre-partal) period and at childbirth may be affected by patriarchal ideology, in which males are valued more than females; a number of Chinese mothers who deliver female babies are more depressed, appear to speak and eat little, sleep a lot, produce less breast milk, care less for their babies, and are usually unwilling to answer questions.

CHAPTER 16
Comprehensive Treatment
综合治疗

WHEN A PREGNANT WOMAN is in critical condition, all doctors should already be thinking of AFE. They are eager to find the specific cause of an illness; however, a patient should first be treated, rather than first being tested, which delays the rescue. One minute may mean the difference between life and death when symptoms are being considered; thus, taking steps to successfully rescue the patient should be the priority. Even if an AFE diagnosis is not clear, treatment should begin immediately to allow for as much time with the patient as possible. In case of imminent danger, emergency measures should begin promptly and contingency plans should be made. The focus of traditional Chinese medicine is to "look, smell, ask, and touch," while the focus of Western medicine is to "look, touch, tap, and listen." I like to use both Chinese and Western medicine. A combination of accurate medical history and diagnostics will help give patients the best treatment. A problem will always have some solution. As Sun Tzu writes in *The Art of War*, "Enemy soldiers can be stopped by generals; water can be soaked up by soil (兵來將擋, 水來土掩)." A doctor should be able to promptly present a wise solution.

Doctors should work to reverse allergic responses, correct respiratory failure, improve hypoxemia, reverse shock, and prevent DIC and renal failure. Treatment should begin for each of the main stages that need to be resolved, step by step. First, the acute shock period should be addressed by increasing oxygen in the blood, and second, the allergic reaction in the pulmonary system should be reversed, using the following information. (1) Oxygen will immediately help maintain airway stability; an endotracheal tube will allow oxygen entry by exerting positive pressure on the airway. If necessary, a tracheotomy should be performed to ensure oxygen entry, reverse alveolar capillary hypoxia, prevent and reduce pulmonary edema, and reverse hypoxia effects to the heart, brain, kidney, and other important organs. (2) To respond to allergic reactions and to reverse hypoxia, large doses of adrenal glucocorticoids should be administered. Antiallergic, antispasmodic drugs will stabilize lysosomes and protect cells. Hydrocortisone, 100–200 mg, should be added to a 5%–10% glucose solution and 50–100 mL administered by rapid intravenous infusion; then, 300–800 mg of hydrocortisone should be added to a 5% glucose solution and 250–500 mL administered by intravenous infusion, at a total daily dose of 500–1000 mg. Alternatively, 20 mg of oral dexamethasone in a 25% glucose solution may be administered by intravenous injection, followed by 20 mg of dexamethasone in a 5%–10% glucose solution administered by intravenous drip. (3) To alleviate pulmonary hypertension, antispasmodic drugs may be administered to improve pulmonary perfusion and prevent respiratory failure due to right heart failure. Papaverine hydrochloride is the drug of choice, administered at a dose of 30–90 mg added to 20 mL of a 10%–25% glucose solution and slowly injected intravenously, with the daily dose not exceeding 300 mg. This treatment will relax smooth muscles, dilate the coronary artery and pulmonary and cerebral arterioles, and reduce the resistance of small blood vessels. Atropine administered at the same time will improve the effect. The atropine dosage is 1 mg in a 10%–25% glucose solution, delivered intravenously in 10 mL volumes every 15 to 30 minutes until the symptoms have subsided. Atropine blocks vagal reflex–induced pulmonary spasm and bronchospasm. A heart rate of >120 beats/min is a signal for cautionary measures to be taken. Aminophylline in the amount of 250 mg added to a 25% glucose solution, injected as a 20 mL bolus, may relax bronchial smooth muscle and relieve pulmonary vasospasm. Phentolamine (Regitine), an alpha-adrenergic inhibitor, in the amount of 5–10 mg in a 10% glucose solution of 100 mL, delivered as an intravenous infusion at a speed of 0.3 mg/min, will relieve pulmonary vasospasm and reduce pulmonary artery resistance and pulmonary hypertension. (4) To treat shock, the blood volume should be replenished. To reverse dilatation, dextran is commonly used in a 400–500 mL intravenous drip, the daily dose not exceeding 1000 mL; it should be added to fresh blood and plasma. The central venous pressure (CVP) should be measured during the rescue effort to inform the doctor of the cardiac load status, thus, the appropriate infusion volume and speed, and a blood sample should be submitted to ascertain the amniotic fluid components.

Drugs to boost blood pressure should also be administered, including oral dopamine, 10–20 mg, in a 10% glucose solution given as an intravenous infusion at a volume of 250 mL. Hydroxylamine, 20–80 mg in a 5% glucose solution intravenously infused, may be used, adjusting the speed according to blood pressure, usually at a drip rate of 20 to 30 drops/min. To correct acidosis, blood oxygen and serum electrolytes should be measured first. If acidosis is present, an intravenous infusion of a 5% sodium bicarbonate solution will correct electrolyte disorders. To correct heart failure, the following drug is commonly used to effect acetylation: Deslanoside, at a dosage of 0.2–0.4 mg, is dissolved in 10% glucose with 20 mL administered by slow delivery intravenously and, if necessary, infused every 4 to 6 hours.

Next, bleeding prevention and DIC control should be addressed: (1) Blood clotting factors should be considered because new blood or plasma, which contains fibrinogen, may be promptly lost. (2) AFE causes an early hypercoagulable state. Heparin, 25–50 mg (1 mg=125 U) in a 0.9% sodium chloride solution, or in 100 mL of a 5% glucose solution, intravenously infused in 1 hour, may be used. In 4 to 6 hours, an additional 50 mg in a 5% glucose solution of 250 mL may be slowly infused. Medication should be controlled during a coagulation time of about 20 to 25 minutes. Heparin, in a total amount of l00–200 mg, may be administered during a 24-hour period. After heparin has been given to the patient, if the clotting time is greater than 30 minutes and there is a bleeding tendency (wound bleeding, postpartum hemorrhage, hematoma, or intracranial hemorrhage), proton antagonism may be used. Protamine, 1 mg, can be used against 100 U of heparin. (3) Anti-fibrinolytic drugs can be administered in the case of hyperfibrinolysis. Aminocaproic acid (4–6 g), ammonia toluic acid

(0.1–0.3 g), or tranexamic acid (0.5–1.0 g) in a 0.9% sodium chloride solution or a 5% glucose solution, intravenously infused in the amount of 100 mL, will inhibit the fibrinolytic enzyme so that plasminogen is not excited, thus inhibiting the dissolution of fibrin. To supplement fibrinogen, administer 2–4 g at a time; a fibrinogen concentration of 1.5 g/L is optimal. (4) Renal failure, which is a third stage of AFE, should be prevented, with urine output being monitored. If oliguria is present, furosemide, 20–40 mg, should be delivered by intravenous injection, or 250 mL of 20% mannitol may be rapidly infused intravenously at a rate of 10 mL/min, to expand the glomerular artery (caution should be used). With renal failure symptoms, blood electrolytes should be monitored. (5) Infection accompanied by nephrotoxicity should be prevented by administering a small dose of broad spectrum antibiotics. (6) If the patient is in the first labor stage, a C-section should be performed to conclude the pregnancy. If the patient is in the second labor stage, the doctor must first make sure that cephalopelvic disproportion and uterine rupture are not present before vaginal delivery can proceed. If postpartum hemorrhaging has begun, hemostasis will not be possible; therefore, a hysterectomy should be performed as quickly as possible to reduce placental dissection and open-sinusoid bleeding. (7) An acupuncturist should take a traditional Chinese medicine approach, using a three-edged needle to puncture (Shi xuan) the tip of each of the 10 fingers, to allow a little bleeding, and ear treatment at the brain and lung points. Electro-acupuncture therapy should be maintained for thirty minutes. The bilateral liver meridian acupuncture point, Tai chong (Liv3), should be used as the sedation method; the acupuncture point on the scalp, Bei hui (GV20), may also be used for sedation. Moxibustion may be used to help relieve AFE symptoms using the point Yong quan (K1), for 15 minutes three times a day. (8) Traditional Chinese medicine for differential treatment uses these herbs: Sheng mai san, Du sheng tang, etc.

CHAPTER 17
Doctor-Patient Cooperation
医患合作

AMNIOTIC FLUID EMBOLISM IS a critical illness, a fatal disorder, and a war against the patient and doctor. Why is the hospital compensated, especially when the doctor does not heal the patient and is then assaulted by the patient's family? Is it possible that doctors are unaware of early detection, preventive measures, diagnosis, the high risks, and mortality rates, and they give the families no clear explanation of AFE? Is it possible that the prenatal education provided is not good enough, as women and their families are presented with no real concept of AFE? Many patients' families think, "We are paying you money, so you must heal the patient. It is not right to pay money to the hospital for the treatment against this hidden killer, when drugs and blood transfusions do not help this patient." As for deciding to perform a C-section, it must not be based on opinions of family members. However, Chinese hospitals require them to sign letters of consent for surgery, although the patients are conscious and can decide for themselves. Family members may be able to authorize decisions for them. Some change has occurred in this policy recently. In principle, Chinese law requires hospitals to compensate families when mistakes are made. If hospitals cannot provide enough evidence to prove they have acted correctly, patients must be compensated. Hospital administration is sometimes poor, reflected in those instances when too few midwives are present to care for the patients, even during the second stage of delivery.

Obstetricians should evaluate some of these issues that occur in the hospital setting. If the family requests a C-section for the patient, the doctor must make a decision, depending on the patient's condition. Doctors may not perform the surgery if childbirth could occur by natural delivery. However, from a legal standpoint, neither family members nor hospitals have the right to make decisions contrary to a mother's wishes; otherwise, they violate civil law. Chenguang Wang, a law professor at Tsinghua University, thinks that doctors should provide patients with detailed scientific analyses that include pros and cons so that they can make their own informed decisions. (春江水暖鸭先知: "When the spring water is warm, the ducks are the first to know.") Mrs. Rongrong, before you jumped from a window, all you needed was a word from your doctor. Could your continuous sharp pain and irritability be an amniotic fluid embolism? Is it possible that your uterine rupture is an omen? (It is estimated that 99% of women who give birth, unless they are Ob-Gyns, do not have knowledge of AFE.) At that point, your Ob-Gyn should quickly drop his or her other work and reexamine you as soon as possible. If the problem is found, your C-section will be given the green light. Your husband, waiting outside, will be quick to sign the agreement for the surgery. You do not need to walk out of the waiting room repeatedly to ask your husband to sign off on the surgery and beg the midwife many times for a C-section. If you ask the questions, the midwife will immediately report to the Ob-Gyn in charge, the attending physician, and the maternity supervisor. Even if you die during C-section, your infant may still be safely delivered. Knowledge is power. If a doctor does not inform a patient about AFE, an innocent child, having already been named by his parents, may be lost because the woman had no knowledge of uterine rupture or other AFE symptoms. That is the main reason for the writing of this book. Doctors, nurses, and patients are warriors in the same trench, fighting side by side to overcome this disorder.

What could be more precious in the world than life? Are there words to describe the feeling of death and loss of a loved one? After such disaster, the families cry out in agony, "Give me back my daughter, my mother, my wife, my family." It is futile to try to get her back. To vent their pain by assaulting the medical staff not only violates the law but also increases the suffering of the family and the medical personnel.

Which career causes a person the greatest pressure? Perhaps no one would disagree that the doctor is under a great amount of stress. According to a recent research report, nearly 80% of doctors have sleep problems and physical diseases. Obstetrics and gynecology, in particular, are unique, busy specialties, at which women in the first, second, and third stages of labor can show up at any time. Ob-Gyns are in effect general practitioners. Because of their great tensions and pressures, doctors and nurses in this field are in a sense like soldiers on a battlefield. While I stood across from the surgeon Dr. Li at an operating table, she suddenly disappeared, her body having slid down onto the floor. It turned out that she had low blood sugar because, being overworked, she had not eaten breakfast. She was often on the job for 24 hours straight, working to save patients through the night. Surgeons at the time often jokingly remarked, "You Ob-Gyns are just like menopausal women."

I saw a report of an AFE death that was followed by a second death. After the AFE death, a competent doctor, emotionally overcome by the painful case, took sleeping pills to commit suicide. It would be unfair to blame doctors and nurses for AFE deaths. I am hopeful that they will begin to see their own selflessness and dedication and end the illogical self-blame. In recent years, a decrease in communication between doctors and patients has occurred in China. Patients no longer have warm feelings for their doctors. Misunderstandings and contradictions have increased, with relationships becoming more tense. Dissatisfaction with the medical profession has spread throughout the society. With assaults and insults against doctors on the rise, the hospital environment has deteriorated and professional honor has declined.

I am hopeful that humankind will come to understand more about this invisible killer, because knowledge is power, and I appeal to the public to be vigilant in the prevention and treatment of AFE. It is hoped that these cases will help raise awareness. Pregnant women must have regular prenatal checkups to allow early detection of problems. Some patients are more aware of abnormal physical changes that take place in their bodies. At the same time, doctors and nurses are very busy and not necessarily able to fully take care of them and detect the abnormal changes. When pregnant women notice such changes, they should take urgent action and not be careless about reporting those changes. Especially in the middle of night, it is easier to overlook changes, miss early detection, and allow the killer to quietly sneak in. Moreover, the disorder will be eerily hidden in a woman's body. In the face of a sudden AFE crisis, a mother and child can remain safe, but this requires the family to trust the doctors and nurses and to cooperate with them, allowing everyone to work together.

CHAPTER 18
The Mystery of the Mona Lisa
名画之谜

CASES OF AMNIOTIC FLUID embolism and maternal mortality occur not only in China but in every corner of the world as well. Scientists and historians are deeply fascinated by the *Mona Lisa*, which was painted in a time that is not too distant from us. They have been working tirelessly with all kinds of high-tech means to try to remove the fog of the *Mona Lisa* that still remains after more than 500 years. Who was the subject of the mystery woman named Mona Lisa? From many researchers, other speculators, and my long-term observation and knowledge of the killer AFE, I have been led to have my own *da Vinci Code* and idea about the *Mona Lisa*.

According to a segment of a CBS Sunday Morning episode televised on October 15, 2017, the mystery behind the smiling woman in Leonardo da Vinci's the *Mona Lisa* has been solved. She was Pacifica Brendano, the girlfriend of Giuliano de Medici, and she died during childbirth, after having given birth to their son. Leonardo's portraits of her were requisitioned to give some peace to the Medici children. A great artist, scientist, and prophet, Leonardo attempted to explain many of the world's mysteries throughout his lifetime. While painting Pacifica's portrait, he must have wondered why she had died during the process of child delivery. What had been the cause? Had her deadly disorder shaped her expression and demeanor?

Why did the painting take four years to complete? Researchers have shown through Leonardo's engravings that he had been studying the killing disorder now known as AFE. Can I conclude without a doubt that Mona Lisa's charming smile is an indication of why she died during the delivery process? Her child lived and was healthy. I have studied Mona Lisa's smile and observed her hair, forehead, eyes, eyebrows, nose, jaws, lip color, and body, and for a long, long time evaluated her form and researched her history. Because of her introverted expression, she is known as the woman with the "mysterious smile." In the portrait, Mona Lisa can be seen to have had a tall figure and a healthy body, but she also had a large pelvis, a slightly anemic face, and a swollen right wrist. Peanut-like nodules protrude from her right hand, near the index finger. I have studied Leonardo's other works, especially paintings and drawings of men and women, and observed no nodules on their hands. There are none similar to the *Mona Lisa*, in which swellings appear on both hands and fingers, and nodules appear on the right hand, near the index finger. Also, there is an especially satirical expression about the eyes and mouth.

In the background of one of the best and earliest copies of the *Mona Lisa* (The Walters Art Museum, Baltimore), the yellow-green color of amniotic fluid is not strong; neither is the vermilion red, which may represent blood. In the copy, the river is not obviously blocked, and the swollen hands and right-hand nodules are not prominent. The water beneath the bridge is green; the overall color is green. After four years of unremitting exploration, wise Leonardo gained a deeper understanding of the disorder that led to the woman's death. In his final masterpiece, which he painted on a poplar panel, he left out the two pillars that were originally part of the background and used predominantly the yellow and green colors of amniotic fluid. The curved river has the look of human blood vessels that have been blocked, and the rapids are the yellowish color of the liver. Mona Lisa's skin and eyes are also yellowish. Even her whole body shows the orange-yellow color of amniotic fluid in the anoxic state of full-term pregnancy.

The landscape of the painting has a deep perspective and is shrouded by a mist similar to the turbidity of amniotic fluid. Features can be recognized that resemble turquoise veins—blocked, diverted blood vessels with extremely curved, serpentine lines—that seem to contain crimson, uncoagulated arterial blood, as would be seen in a pregnant woman with AFE. Behind Mona Lisa, the land moves up and down in a disorganized way. Ferocious greens, yellows, grays, and whites may represent a hurricane-like pouring of amniotic fluid into the woman's body. A red color is used in the background, as if the woman is lying in a pool of blood. The hue is similar to the deep pink, cinnabar-red color of arterial blood. The greenish color around the river may represent the effect of carbon monoxide during hypoxia. Also, the same vermilion-red color can be seen that I saw during the rescue of a woman with AFE, whose uncoagulated blood flowed from her vagina.

Once Leonardo had painted Medici's girlfriend, why not give the painting to the client instead of keeping it around? And why did he name this riddle of a portrait the *Mona Lisa*? Perhaps *Mona* represents the male, and *Lisa*, the female. My theory is that *Mona* and *Lisa* represent a portrait of the killer who embodied the child born after the union of the yin and yang. The background clearly depicts the yellow-green color of a full-term fetus after anal sphincter relaxation and discharge of meconium-stained amniotic fluid. The background is less red than green. The bridge in the rear may be an omen, a prediction of the arrival of the tangible material in the fluid resulting from the disorder, caused by microthrombosis. Mona Lisa's swollen right wrist and fingers and the bump near her thumb and index finger suggest that her body was affected by fluid exudation and blockage.

As an expert at the autopsy table and in human anatomy, I have observed the death scene and reached a conclusion. Doctors are expert at spotting problems from the outside and the inside and can recognize diseases on the face based on ancient Chinese physiognomy. I can see that Mona Lisa was not only beautiful but was also previously healthy and only slightly anemic. She may have died during childbirth for many reasons. Perhaps serious complications caused her to have the pulmonary embolism, shock, and DIC that led to her death. My speculation is that she most likely died after postpartum hemorrhage because of AFE. Of course, we should continue to explore this mystery.

The dear Mona Lisa, young and mysterious, was diminished at a most beautiful moment in her life. It was not she who failed. Rather, possibly, she was killed by the disorder called amniotic fluid embolism. Her enigmatic beauty remains for future generations to contemplate. Perhaps her mysterious expression actually reflects the killer's smile! Did the intelligent Leonardo da Vinci convey the killer's message to the world 513 years ago?

Amniotic fluid embolism was first discovered by the medical profession in 1941. If AFE is revealed to be Mona Lisa's killer, and Leonardo da Vinci's original intention was to show us that, then we will have guessed his password, and thus the world will be less entangled and less suspicious. (潮平兩岸闊, 風正一帆懸: "When the winds are calm, the tides are low on both sides of the river; with a fair wind, only a single sail is needed.") At the same time, we can deeply salute the great man who was also a great artist and scientist. By the way, during the Renaissance, the great Leonardo da Vinci first described the existence of the mesentery of the human body, but it was ignored throughout the centuries. We medical experts did not officially recognize this double fold of the peritoneum—the lining of the abdominal cavity—that holds the intestine to the wall of the abdomen until October 2016, when it was described in the prestigious journal *The Lancet*. The mesentery is listed as the 79th organ of the human body.

CHAPTER 19
In the Future
继往开来

AMNIOTIC FLUID EMBOLISM, REGARDLESS of national boundaries, origin, religion, poverty, or wealth, may visit any woman who is pregnant or about to become a mother. Whether she is beautiful or ordinary, whether she lives in the desert of Ningxia City, or near the beautiful blue Danube in Austria, whether during childbirth the woman's husband is on patrol in a nuclear submarine in the depths of the sea, or still guards her bedside, AFE may wander in the atmosphere around her during her pregnancy. It does not matter whether the man carries a powerful weapon or farm tools, or whether the woman is a millionaire, a middle-class woman, or a woman who needs financial support. AFE, like a feather floating in midair, may appear in someone's body. Similar events are often reported around the world, ringing the alarm bells for us again and again. In the US and England, there are dedicated foundations that provide financial and psychological help to patients and their families who suffer from AFE. It is my hope that China will set up one as well. We must try to help people avoid suffering helplessly and also provide psychological counseling to medical staff, who are secondary victims. We must try to get out of the shadow of the killer AFE. The well-being of women should be placed in a higher position, enabling future generations to be safer and healthier. Cooperation by doctors and patients and their families is necessary. The stars have continued shining over the vast history of human civilization, during space travel and ocean exploration (可上九天揽月, 可下五洋捉鳖) and the advancement of the Internet, science, and technology, including biological engineering and artificial intelligence development. It is recommended that we study AFE using nanotechnology. Where there's a will, there's a way. Medicine is the gateway to the natural sciences and can be used to find the truth, the correct understandings, and solutions to problems. Instead of letting the facts be covered up, we should not allow the killer to continue maiming mothers and then disappearing "outside the law." Our goals are high, so we must continue to work hard in the future. Doctors should try to prevent disorders like AFE, tactically defying the enemy's strategy—with the emphasis on *enemy* (不战而屈人之兵: "Beat the enemy without fighting."). If doctors are not prepared for battle, AFE will win, as it has no internal strife to contend with. This world can defeat this killer of pregnant women. On this note, I wish everyone—and their families and friends—good luck, good health, happiness, and blessings!

THE END

Bitao Lian

REFERENCES

1. Zheng Huai Mei, Su Ying Kuan, Eds. *Obstetrics and Gynecology*, 2nd Ed., Higher Medical Colleges Teaching Materials, People's Health Publishing House, Beijing.

2. Xie Xing, Gou Wenli. *Obstetrics and Gynecology*, 8th Ed., People's Health Publishing House, Beijing, March 2013, pp. 215-218.

3. Le Jie. *Obstetrics and Gynecology*, 7th Ed., People's Health Publishing House, Beijing, 2007, pp. 208-210.

4. Zhang Dan, Yang Shaoping, Zhang Bin, Yang Rong, Mei Hui. Analysis of maternal mortality due to amniotic fluid embolism in Wuhan from 2001 to 2014, Chinese Maternal and Child Health Care, 2006, 31(3):475-477.

5. Pantaleo G, Luigi N, Federica T, et al. Amniotic fluid embolism: review, Curr Pharm Biotechnol, 2014, 14(14):1163-1167.

6. McDonnell NJ, Percival V, Paech MJ. Amniotic fluid embolism: a leading cause of maternal death yet still a medical conundrum, Int J Obstet Anesth, 2013, 22(4):329-336.

7. Pacheco LD, Saade G, Hankins GD, et al. Fluid embolism: diagnosis and management, Am J Obstet Gynecol, Aug. 2016, 215(2):B16-24.

AFTERWORD
掩卷

IT IS MY FIRM intention to keep learning and cultivating, enriching, and improving myself. I am wholeheartedly inspired to unify my knowledge and practice. I work to develop the highest technical skills, and I feel true compassion for my patients. It is my lifelong goal to always work for their benefit and to win their trust and support.

– Bitao Lian, Christmas Eve, 2017, in Gainesville, Florida, USA

Made in the USA
Columbia, SC
09 November 2024

45904207R00070